STUCK
IN TIME

ALSO BY LEE GUTKIND

Bike Fever

The Best Seat in Baseball, But You Have to Stand

God's Helicopter (a novel)

The People of Penn's Woods West

Our Roots Grow Deeper Than We Know

Many Sleepless Nights

One Children's Place

STUCK IN TIME

The Tragedy of
Childhood Mental Illness

LEE GUTKIND

Henry Holt and Company
New York

Henry Holt and Company, Inc.
Publishers since 1866
115 West 18th Street
New York, New York 10011

Henry Holt® is a registered trademark
of Henry Holt and Company, Inc.

Published in Canada by Fitzhenry & Whiteside Ltd.,
195 Allstate Parkway, Markham, Ontario L3R 4T8.

Library of Congress Cataloging-in-Publication Data
Gutkind, Lee.
Stuck in time : the tragedy of childhood mental
illness / Lee Gutkind.—1st ed.
p.   cm.
1. Adolescent psychiatry—United States—Case studies.
2. Teenagers—Mental health services—United States—Case studies.
3. Teenagers—Mental health services—United States.
4. Mentally ill children—United States—Case studies. I. Title.
RJ503.G88   1993   92-45087
616.89´022—dc20   CIP

ISBN 0-8050-1469-1
ISBN 0-8050-3808-6 (An Owl Book: pbk.)

Henry Holt books are available for special promotions
and premiums. For details contact: Director, Special Markets.

First published in hardcover in 1993 by
Henry Holt and Company, Inc.

First Owl Book Edition—1995

Designed by Katy Riegel

Printed in the United States of America
All first editions are printed on acid-free paper.∞

1   3   5   7   9   10   8   6   4   2
1   3   5   7   9   10   8   6   4   2
(pbk.)

This book is dedicated to Mrs. Duncan, who died recently after forty years of voluntary service. No one loved children, revered families, or spent herself more vehemently on their behalf.

Author's Note

Parents, such as Tom and Elizabeth Scanlon, who have children with mental health problems, are often forced into untenable, desperate situations because of a lack of options and not because of a lack of love. I observed the Scanlons and other families in similar situations for nearly three years. Despite their struggles, I never doubted the love and commitment they shared.

In certain cases, pseudonyms have been used to protect confidentiality. However, all the people who appear in this book are real, as are their stories.

Contents

Acknowledgments

Ronald E. Dahl, M.D., has engaged with me in a continuously probing dialogue about children with mental health problems and the challenges and complications of scientific research. He painstakingly examined *Stuck in Time* with a keen and critical eye that helped shape the final product.

Jane Knitzer's book *Unclaimed Children*, published by the Children's Defense Fund in 1982, first uncovered the inequities faced by children with mental health problems and their families. Dr. Knitzer's editorial recommendations were invaluable. Her encouragement was inspiring.

When I decided to reverse the direction of this book as originally proposed, Bill Strachan, my editor, trusted me. Bill's faith and patience are rare and vital attributes.

Western Psychiatric Institute and Clinic provided remarkable and mostly unfettered access. The social workers, physicians, psychologists, nurses, milieu therapists, administrators, and support personnel with whom I came into contact were always cooperative. The librarians at Western Psych's film and video section were especially diligent and resourceful on my behalf.

The National Mental Health Association (NMHA) was unfailingly responsive to my requests for information, vital statistics, and expert referrals. With Tipper Gore and Ann Simpson as co-chairs, the NMHA organized the Child Mental Health Interest Group, a nonpartisan group of spouses of current and former members of Congress, which sponsored an invaluable series of educational activities in 1990–91, helping to build support for children and families at the highest levels of government.

Give Families a Break (GFAB), organized by United Mental Health, Inc., of Western Pennsylvania, gave passionate assistance. The Parents Involved Network (PIN), the American Psychiatric Association, the American Academy of Child and Adolescent Psychiatry, the National Institute of Mental Health, and the National Alliance of the Mentally Ill all provided vital information.

I would also like to express appreciation for financial support from The Freedom Forum's Publication Program for Journalists in Education and its founder, Professor James Carey.

I conducted more than a hundred interviews for *Stuck in Time* and spent countless hours with the people described in these pages in a variety of locations. In addition to those included in the book or named above, I would also like to thank Patt Franciossi, Gina White, Chris Koyanagi, Neal Ryan, David Kupfer, Beverly Aleo, Beverly Milofsky, Gary Pletsch, Lila Decker, Carol Anderson, John Campo, Richard Cohen, Robert Tetter, Jess Amchin, Judy Warwzeniak, Susan McPheeters, Joseph Strayhorn, Joachim Puig Antich, Michael Rancurello, Katherine Wisner, Walter Kaye, Rolf Loeber, Mary Margaret Kerr, Jim Volano, Fred Fowler, Marcus Kruesi, Judith Rappaport, Peter Jensen, Peter Tanguay, Heidi Friend, Cindy Smith, Manuel Garcia, Victor Papale, Cheryl Kubelik, Michael Strober, Edwin Ritvo, Mark DeAntonio, Robert Dealy, Ronna Harris, Ruth Drescher, Richard Simmons, Bonnie Zima, Anne Spence, Glenda Fine, Connie Dellmuth, and Patricia Park, as well as Carole Kunkle-Miller, whose twelve-year-old patient is responsible for the original art for the book jacket, and Raquel Jaramillo, its designer.

Preface

As I worked on this book, I periodically thought about a scene in Kurt Vonnegut's novel *Slaughterhouse-Five*. The protagonist Billy Pilgrim entered his living room, turned on the television, and suddenly became "slightly unstuck in time," an event that enabled him to watch the late movie—an epic about American bomber pilots in World War II—backward. This was a marvelously therapeutic experience: American planes, riddled with bullet holes and bloodied men, took off from an English airfield backward, and flew backward to France, where they were confronted by German fighters, which sucked bullets back into gun barrels protruding from their cockpits. The Americans followed the fighters to Germany, backward, where fire and debris were siphoned up from the earth into big bombs. As the backward procession continued, the bombs were stacked on racks in England, then transported on ships to the U.S., where American pilots were transformed into high school kids. The movie subsequently reversed direction, but Billy Pilgrim speculated that if the backward momentum had continued, Adolf Hitler might have been a baby and Adam and Eve reborn.

This is what I wish for the three children—Daniel, Meggan, and Terri—whose stories I chronicle here; that somehow, with the flick of a switch or the wave of a magic wand, they too might become "unstuck in time," triggering a journey backward to their own hopeful beginnings, thus launching a new and better start in life, not only for them, but for all the 7.5 to 9.5 million U.S. children who suffer from serious mental health problems. Four fifths of those children receive no treatment, while even the "lucky" remaining minority are often treated inappropriately.

Researching and writing this book, I met many intelligent and compassionate people: the personnel at Western Psychiatric Institute and Clinic (Western Psych), where I regularly observed treatments; the national child mental health care experts I interviewed; the psychiatrist Kenneth Stanko, who welcomed me into his inner sanctum. They, like the families and kids they are dedicated to protecting and treating, are also *stuck in time*, mired in an outdated and overextended system that only infrequently functions therapeutically for anybody.

Kurt Vonnegut's work reflects a unique understanding of the absurdity of a system and situation that so blatantly defy logic. Perhaps new leaders will emerge to help improve child mental health care in the U.S., but at present our best bet for salvation and change is the immediate re-creation of Billy Pilgrim, who can reverse our senseless direction.

STUCK
IN TIME

DANIEL

Autumn

WHEN I DROVE up to the house, Daniel was walking toward me. I got
out of the car and waited for him to approach. Even though he waved
and flashed a quick smile, he seemed grim and befuddled. "What's
wrong, Dan?"

He shrugged and shook his head as we walked up the steps toward
the porch. "Nothing's wrong," he said, but his eyes were darting erratically from side to side.

Daniel had been working periodically that summer at a rental property I owned, cleaning out the basement, a filthy job that he savored.
Nothing made Daniel happier than getting dirty, especially with a
bunch of junk. A pack rat, Daniel had always rummaged through trash,
rescuing an array of worthless mechanical objects—manual typewriters,
speedometers, radios, lamps, rusty tools, old motors. Keys of any size,
type, or condition were his special passion, and locks, whether or not
they corresponded to the keys. Sometimes he managed to clean or fix a
derelict item of junk and sell it at a Sunday flea market, but usually
Daniel was more interested in contemplating these items in the questionable safety of his room.

Daniel is short and broad, part muscle from his recent forays into
weight lifting and part paunch from overeating. It was not unusual for

him to devour an entire large pizza with mushrooms, sausage, and pepperoni—our traditional Saturday-afternoon snack—followed by a few hot sausage hoagies for dinner. Over the past three years, he had changed a good deal physically; when he was twelve, he weighed ninety pounds, a frail and exceedingly delicate feather of a boy; now, still very short, he could be more aptly described as a fireplug.

We stopped at the top of the steps, and I put my hands on his shoulders. Ruffling his curly hair with my hand, I joked about how dirty he was and made a crack about his ears, which are unusually small. I could almost always get him to laugh by invoking his ears or by pointing out that he was most handsome on Halloween, when he wore a mask. But this time he did not laugh, or protest; he was so somber that I pulled him down on the stoop and looked him straight in the eye. "C'mon Dan. Something's wrong. What's going on?"

Although I could see it coming, I was surprised at the power of his emotions. A mask of fear suddenly exploded onto his face, and he began to whine, like a small, frightened child. "Oh, I'm so scared," he said. "He's going to kill me."

His eyes darted crazily, and he tried to stand up and run, but I held on to him. "I won't let anyone hurt you."

Tears were streaming down his face, which he buried in my chest. "A man molested me." He reached down and began squeezing his buttocks. "Oh, it hurts," he wailed. "It hurts so bad back there."

Daniel poured out his story in the midst of choking sobs. He had worked in the basement for half an hour or so, dragging out a mess of discarded timber, empty paint cans, and old furniture, and then decided to take a five-minute walk to the local convenience store for a soda. There's a bank of pay phones on the corner beside the store, and as he was passing, a phone was ringing. Daniel answered. A male voice at the other end said that he had been waiting for Daniel and would kill him if he didn't do what he was told. "Yeah, sure," Daniel had replied, hanging up the phone and going to the store.

But when Daniel walked past the telephones on his return, a car screeched to a halt at the curb. A man, unshaven, dressed in black trousers and shirt and black patent leather shoes and waving a knife, ordered Daniel inside. Instead of running, or screaming—or even laughing—Daniel complied. They drove around the corner, down a side street, and into an alley, whereupon the man led Daniel through a clump of bushes behind an abandoned building. Following orders, Daniel kissed the man on the lips, then, under threat of the knife, sank to his knees and performed oral sex. Finally, Daniel lay facedown on the ground. The man entered him. Daniel felt a sharp and intrusive pain. Now, at the end of the story, Daniel was nearly hysterical. "Oh, it hurts so bad. He said he'd kill me if I told anyone. What am I going to do?"

I could not answer his question, for I felt dumbfounded and conflicted. This incident had occurred in my neighborhood, an area in which I lived with my wife and infant son, and one considered the most urbane in the city. Not that crime never occurred here, but child molestation (or kidnapping) in the middle of a bright and busy Saturday afternoon was unlikely, to say the least.

Besides, there was Daniel's history to consider, beginning with the abuse and neglect that had led authorities to permanently separate Daniel from his family when he was ten years old. The abuse during his early years had been documented, but recently, new and questionable incidents of violence and molestation had allegedly occurred. Only a couple of weeks ago, Daniel had come home with his face bruised and his books and wallet missing. He claimed to have been attacked by four black kids, wielding pipes, who stole his money and beat him up. Later, witnesses reported that he had actually gotten into a fight with a neighborhood kid, who was white—and lost.

Last year, Daniel had reported that a teenage female resident of his group home had accosted him in a darkened passageway and molested him. At about the same time, Daniel told a convoluted story about being followed by a mysterious bearded man who had forced him into his Cadillac and molested him. Daniel also claimed that a teacher at school was abusing him and encouraging him to run away and not attend classes.

Many of the past horrors in Daniel's life had been confirmed, but his recent credibility was partially suspect because of his own maliciousness. Hadn't he, one Saturday afternoon, removed all the manhole covers from the sewer system on the periphery of his group home and covered the holes with twigs, grass, and weeds as "booby traps"? Hadn't he promised, after I had explained the danger, to immediately replace the manhole covers, and hadn't he reneged on that promise? Didn't he lie frequently about where he went and what he did, using his learning disabilities and the side effects from antidepressant medication as justifications for forgetting and making mistakes?

Some of his excuses were plausible, especially those attributed to his learning disabilities. The intent of messages directed toward him sometimes did not register, but because Daniel was intuitive and responsive, he skillfully maintained eye contact with the person to whom he was speaking, able to sense when to shake his head, shrug, or nod, indicating understanding while completely in the dark. But there was an unpredictable side to Daniel, as well; he was a kid who tottered on the precarious edge of ambiguity.

The "booby trap" incident had been especially disturbing because it made me realize that Daniel's defensiveness could distort his sense of right and wrong. The caseworker at his group home observed that Daniel had been so brutally battered by his family and by the child welfare system that "rescued" him that it was impossible for him to feel compassion. The fact that someone could have been hurt—or killed—by his "booby traps" meant little to Daniel, who frequently declared, "I don't care about anyone else."

I don't believe that Daniel wants to hurt anyone, but because of his history, he possesses an irrational and uncontrollable fear of being taken advantage of, especially by someone unknown. This helps to explain his penchant for locks, keys, and burglar alarms, and suspicions toward strangers. Daniel could have seen this unshaven man dressed in black sitting in his car or making a telephone call and his imagination might have done the rest.

Daniel continued to whimper as I tried to decide how to proceed. At the very least, I had to get him away from this house and the fear that the mysterious man, whether real or imagined, was going to come back for him. I remembered a story he'd told me of another unshaven man who lived in the woods across from his home who would periodically sneak into the room he occupied with his sister—and molest them both. The power of his emotions and the horror of what might have happened to him confused and frightened me. Hurriedly, we gathered his possessions and climbed into my car.

I drove in the general direction of the convenience store until Daniel pointed to the street to which the man had taken him. Instinctively, I turned the corner, Daniel directing me into the alley he had described. For the first time, I began to believe that the incident could have happened. The alley was not dark or narrow, but it was clearly out of the way, as was the building to which he pointed, set off in a secluded corner of a vacant lot. The underbrush around the building was thick and concealing. If a molestation had occurred, it could have happened here.

I backed down the alley and once again headed for the store. A police van was sitting in the parking lot, its engines idling. Out of the corner of my eye, I could see two officers, both women, eating a take-out lunch and listening to their walkie-talkie. Daniel was staring straight ahead, whimpering and snuffling. He did not see the police van, but its presence provided a direction—right or wrong.

"Well, Dan, this is your chance," I said, pointing at the white van with its large blue-and-gold official seal. "We could approach those officers and tell them what happened."

Daniel did not hesitate. "Yes," he said, with conviction. Daniel has always possessed an irrepressible penchant for law enforcement officers, which is what he wanted to become. The order and control that police may establish appeals to kids who have lacked the order and control which might have made their lives happier and safer. As Daniel had grown older, the idea of being a policeman had faded, although their uniforms and authority were still quite seductive.

We got out of the car, walked across the parking lot, and knocked on the window of the van. "I was molested by a man dressed in black," Daniel said. He quickly highlighted the gruesome details.

Almost instantly, the officer on the driver's side activated her walkie-talkie. Announcing the specific location, I heard her summarize Daniel's story to her sergeant, using the word that both Daniel and I had studiously avoided: "A reported rape . . ."

Within five minutes, the entire parking lot was ringed with police vehicles. Daniel was asked to tell his story twice more, once by a sergeant and then by a medic, and with each telling Daniel became more distraught. He buried his face in my chest and began sobbing uncontrollably, especially when the medic attempted to take him in the ambulance to the hospital for the long and intense physical examination required.

"Lee, you have to come with me; I don't want to be alone."

"You go in the ambulance, Dan. I'll be along in my own car. Don't worry, I won't leave you."

When I arrived at the emergency room a few minutes later, the police would not permit me to join him in the examination room; Daniel remained alone with the doctors, nurses, and policemen for the next six hours. As directed, I went home and sat by the telephone, waiting for the police to contact me. I did not know what to believe—or even what I wanted to believe. Did I want the police to determine that Daniel was telling the truth—that he had really been raped? Or would it be preferable to learn that Daniel had been lying or hallucinating? Either way, Daniel was the ultimate victim—of society, his family, his biology, and of himself.

PART ONE

The Scanlons

1

I FIRST LEARNED of Tom and Elizabeth Scanlon from Debbie Rubin when she and I met for coffee one afternoon in the cafeteria of Western Psychiatric Institute and Clinic ("Western Psych" to Pittsburghers), part of the University of Pittsburgh Medical Center. Rubin, a social worker on the Adolescent Affective (Mood) Disorders Unit, 3 West, had just completed a family therapy session with Tom and Elizabeth and their fifteen-year-old daughter, Meggan, which she described as "the saddest meeting I have ever heard." Elizabeth was at her wits' end, sobbing hysterically, and then Meggan read excerpts of the personal journal patients are required to keep. "She began to cry and then Tom began to cry. I cried, too," said Rubin. "Elizabeth and Tom are going through a mourning process—mourning the loss of who they had dreamed their daughter would be."

I asked Debbie if I could meet the Scanlons. I had been observing on 3 West for about six months, during which time I had come to realize that facilities like Western Psych, although scientifically renowned, attracted a large majority of disadvantaged children, adolescents, and adults. For a variety of reasons, poor people are more apt to be victims of mental disorders from the earliest ages.

In a 1989 report, *Research on Children and Adolescents with Mental, Behavioral and Developmental Disorders*, the Institute of Medicine (IOM) identified nine primary factors leading to mental illness in children, many directly related to the family's socioeconomic position. These include biological insults, such as physical trauma or exposure to toxic chemicals (lead poisoning) or drugs; poor prenatal care, resulting in a high risk of prematurity; persistent environmental adversity, such as poverty, inadequate schools, or homelessness; abuse and neglect; and disturbed family relationships. Indirectly related are causes that include chronic physical illness, such as leukemia, diabetes, epilepsy, and AIDS; cognitive impairments such as those resulting from mental retardation and deficits in sensory perception, including blindness and deafness; parental mental illness, with the accompanying and often traumatic disruptions of family life; and basic genetic factors that increase a child's vulnerability to a host of mood and anxiety disorders.

Though poverty is often a precursor to mental illness, middle-class families with children who have emotional problems must consume many of their resources before they receive child welfare support. The Scanlons had exhausted their savings, as well as the equity in their home, and had gone $42,000 into debt in order to provide special education and counseling for Meggan, their younger son, Doug, and themselves.

Even more perplexing to the Scanlons was the fact that after all this time and effort from pediatricians, psychiatrists, and psychologists, no one could say with certainty what was wrong with Meggan—why she acted the way she did—or, more important how to control or modify her behaviors. Theories about Meggan's diagnosis and treatment were plentiful, but successful solutions had not been forthcoming. Equally dismaying was the fact that some people, friends and family members particularly, actually doubted that Meggan was mentally ill, attributing her behaviors to normal childhood development and/or poor parenting. And it was entirely possible that Tom and Elizabeth had significantly contributed to Meggan's downfall—the puzzle of mental illness is convoluted and intertwined.

THE SCANLONS ARE an engaging and youthful couple, both in their early forties. Tom is of medium height, with brown hair neatly combed to the side, and a rough, reddish complexion. For a while, he lived in Johnstown, Pennsylvania, the coal-country town of 20,000 where the popular Paul Newman movie about minor league hockey, *Slap Shot*, was filmed. Tom's parents were strict and authoritarian, and Tom's inability to discipline his daughter, as did his parents their son, has been a source of conflict for both sides of the family. He is disciplined about himself, though, watching his diet, keeping physically fit. In 1990, he ran the Marine Corps Marathon in Washington, D.C., in a respectable three and a half hours. As an accountant who serves as liaison between his employer, Westinghouse Electric Company, and the Internal Revenue Service, he is patient, down-to-earth, and always congenial.

At first meeting, Elizabeth is more extroverted. She recently earned an undergraduate degree with a major in sociology and minor in creative writing "so that I could capture our exciting adventures with Meggan," she says with a nervous but hearty laugh. She laughs often, with disconcerting spontaneity, while describing some of her worst moments as a parent. Her sudden bursts of humor in unfunny situations sometimes seem surreal.

Her father was a faculty member at Pennsylvania State University, and her maternal grandfather's name was Millard Fillmore Kidney. "There have been many people in our family with the same name, and we are definitely related, although this is not a source of pride or satisfaction." The laughter erupts again, revealing a row of small, straight teeth. "What can you say about a man—even a former President of the United States—who was elected to office on the 'Know Nothing' party ticket?"

The Scanlons live in Mt. Lebanon, a well-to-do Pittsburgh suburb with a school district recognized for excellence, producing more National Merit Scholars than most other districts of its size in the nation. "We're an old-style family," Meggan told me, "but we have lots of fun. Everybody has a lot in common. When people argue, it is about stupid things. My parents get along really wonderfully. We live in a house where the outside looks like a modern home but the inside is all decorated with country stuff."

In a way, the Scanlons' life is also much different on the outside, in that it resembles a comfortable suburban family existence, compared to the gauntlet of suffering endured within. When she wants to be—and especially with strangers and adults—Meggan is incredibly charming.

After Meggan was interviewed for an exclusive private school, her parents asked the admissions counselor if she would be accepted, to which he replied: "If she wanted to, she could be elected vice-president of AT&T."

In addition to caring for Meggan and Douglas, thirteen, Elizabeth works full time as a business consultant/office manager for a group of orthopedic surgeons in private practice and part time as a student. "The worst day of my life was when I graduated college. There were no more classes to attend. I immediately moved into graduate study and the work force because I could not bear the thought of coming home and facing Meggan." Escape has been a primary motivation almost from Meggan's birth.

"I remember a very special weekend," says Tom. "We got Elizabeth's sister to watch the kids, and we came to Pittsburgh, shacked up in a hotel, went to movies and dinner. Driving back was the worst I had ever seen Elizabeth. She literally cried the entire way, because she was returning to Meggan. How she's lasted this long is beyond me." He persuaded her to put the children in a day-care center and find a job.

"Meggan liked the structure of the day-care center," Tom continued. "She liked having other kids to play with and planned activities. But all that stuff dries up when you get to be a teenager, and that's when all the serious problems started. She just got out of control. Elizabeth kept saying, 'Maybe I should quit my job and stay home.' But I resisted. 'In a matter of six weeks, you'll be in a nuthouse.' "

Outside the home, Elizabeth's friends "identify me as being a mover, somebody in control: 'If you want something done, ask Elizabeth.' Inside my house I am like dirt on the floor that my daughter grinds into the rug. Her rhetoric can crush me. Meggan takes a razor blade to my psyche. My daughter can make my life miserable; she rips me to shreds."

Tom and Elizabeth were very open with me; one might almost say *anxious* to talk to me because, I think, hardly anyone except social workers fulfilling the responsibilities of their profession ever listened to them. *Real* people—family, friends, and neighbors—were not particularly responsive. Elizabeth's family had problems of its own, so they couldn't always be bothered by Elizabeth's concerns. Tom's family was convinced that Meggan had not been properly disciplined, which was the reason for her bizarre and oppositional behavior. What she needed was "a good kick in the butt to knock some sense into her."

Friends discounted Meggan's actions with comparisons to those of their own children. If Elizabeth said Meggan screamed at the top of her lungs for hours, they would reply, "You should hear my daughter when she's angry." If Elizabeth complained that Meggan stayed up half the night or walked uninvited into their bedroom and stared until she or Tom opened their eyes, friends would say, "All children have trouble with sleep," or, "She's only an impetuous teenager; give her time to grow up." But the Scanlons had been giving Meggan time and monumental effort from the day she was born.

Meggan Scanlon was a different sort of baby from the moment she entered the world. At the hospital nursery, Meggan alienated the nurses by waking all the other babies and upsetting their feeding schedule with her constant crying. At home, she was skittish and volatile, overly sensitive to light, noise, any stimulation. "She just didn't seem real happy, and she was hitting herself, angry all the time," said Elizabeth. "She was in the hospital emergency room constantly. She broke her leg when she was three, and she was constantly falling on her face. She sustained a second-degree burn from a grow light. She took a razor and shaved off her lip. She shoved a button up her nose. She drank prescription medicine, set fire to her bedroom. There were gates all over the house."

What confounded the Scanlons was their inability to exercise any control. "When she was four years old, not yet potty trained, she learned how to take her diapers off. We used the cloth diapers, and she was able to unpin them, but couldn't put them back on. At night, she would call us to her room to show how creative she had been, being able to take her diaper off. We told her, 'You can't do that, Meggan; you're going to lie here in bed for the whole night in a puddle of water.' We put the diaper back on, but the next night, 'Mom, Dad.' She'd got it off again. We spanked her, but it made no difference.

"Every night she would announce with glee that she had taken her diaper off. Every night. By the end of the second week, we looked at each other—we were both shaking—and decided to stop fighting. She would never give up. No way. As the years passed, we finally recognized that Meggan always resists. You could absolutely beat Meggan to death and she would not give in or stop fighting."

During Meggan's first four years, the Scanlons changed pediatricians five times. One pediatrician maintained that they were facing the normal challenges of child-rearing. Bringing up the child was a war and you had to plan your battles and win when you could. Another pediatrician at a local child-guidance center in Pittsburgh provided a name for Meggan's problem. "She's temperamentally difficult," the doctor concluded after listening to a description of Meggan's oppositional behavior.

"This was the first time anyone had actually acknowledged that it was not our parenting at fault," said Tom, "that we had a problem child. We were almost weeping with joy because it wasn't us. We looked at the doctor and asked how to treat a 'temperamentally difficult' child. That's when he said, 'You're in for a life of misery. There's nothing anybody can do.'"

"He wouldn't even meet Meg," Elizabeth interrupted. "He wouldn't reappoint us." His only contribution was to direct the Scanlons to the Child Development Unit at Pittsburgh's Children's Hospital. The Scanlons were invited to join a parent support group which met once a week and to take part in behavior modification training sessions. Many of the approaches and techniques were effective for a "honeymoon period," a few weeks of euphoria when they believed they had discovered a way of reaching and controlling Meggan, but none—stars on the wall or money in the bank as incentives, special privileges for special behavior—was self-sustaining.

There was some solace, however, in being with other parents who were enduring similarly frustrating and confusing challenges with their own children. "You're almost afraid to meet other people in the same boat because you think something's got to be wrong with them. And if something's wrong with them, then it stands to reason something's wrong with you," said Tom. "But the others were nice and normal. We cared a lot about our kids."

Eventually the Scanlons entered family therapy with Dr. William Cohen, a developmental pediatrician, the theory being that the entire family had to learn to deal with Meggan since changing Meggan's behavior did not seem to be in the cards. Family therapy was useful in that "it kept us married," said Elizabeth, "because people do tend to blame each other in child-rearing situations." But as far as dealing with Meggan, the best the Scanlons could achieve was a series of honeymoon periods followed by dashed hopes. It was an inescapably vicious circle.

By the time she was thirteen, Meggan had discovered sex and was becoming promiscuous. Her interest in boys was obsessive; in public, she would seek out the most appealing male in the room—sometimes someone twice her age—and encourage him, sometimes with Elizabeth and Tom observing. A twenty-seven-year-old man she had approached pursued her home from the library one day; the boy Meggan had befriended at a campground during a summer vacation wanted the family to bring their camper to his house on New Year's Eve to shoot off their guns. "He called us regularly for years, and we would tell him not to call back—but Meggan insisted on phoning him," said Elizabeth. Meggan approached a whole range of characters. "She goes up to people in wheelchairs and asks what's wrong with their legs.

"You just never know what to expect. I was thinking the other day about that English teacher who asked Meggan to take a test. Meggan refused and cursed her out. The teacher said, 'I bet your mother would have something to say if she knew the way you were behaving.' And Meggan told her, 'No, my mother allows me to talk like this.'

"So the woman called me at home that night and said, 'In thirty years of teaching, no one has ever spoken to me the way your daughter did. And she said you don't mind.' I said, 'Give me a break. Of course I mind. That couldn't be farther from the truth.' We are horrified by her ongoing behaviors because we have been her favorite victims."

Meggan would often telephone her parents and ask them to pick her up, but when they arrived at the appointed time and place, she would not be there. Once they were to meet at a local park. "We looked everywhere. We went around the block. We hiked the trails. We phoned people she knew. The early evening turned to the pitch black of night, and we felt as if we were living a nightmare. I finally said to Tom, 'We have no choice. We have to call the police.' All the while, I couldn't stop thinking about what people would say. I had this vision of myself on the eleven o'clock news, holding a picture of Meggan and facing a reporter demanding: 'Aren't you her mother? Don't you know where she is supposed to be?' And there I am, the most irresponsible, complete failure of a parent since the beginning of time, without any answers." Tom eventually found Meggan exactly where she had promised to meet them. "According to Meggan, she had been there all the time—waiting for us."

In most matters, Meggan was generally unreliable. Whatever time she promised to come home after school or meeting a friend was disregarded without a moment's hesitation. When confronted, Meggan would lie, often making up conflicting stories to satisfy whatever questions Tom, Elizabeth, or her teachers might ask. It did not seem to matter that everyone knew she was lying—Meggan would defend herself with indignant passion. When it became inescapably evident that she was at fault, Meggan would suddenly become contrite and apologetic, admitting guilt, assuming responsibility, and suggesting severe punishments to compensate for her behavior. Meggan would agree to any punishment; it didn't matter, for she refused to comply with any of them. Meggan passionately resisted any attempt to control her life.

Meggan's actions also had a devastating effect on her younger brother—Douglas suffered from attention deficit hyperactivity disorder (ADHD). His therapist told Tom and Elizabeth that he "gunnysacked," meaning that he suppressed his feelings, until suddenly his fury would explode. In art therapy, "he drew bleeding decapitated animals, reptiles, humans," Elizabeth said.

"The doctors said that we should try to keep the kids apart as much as possible." Doug and Meggan could not be trusted at home alone for a sustained period because it would "initiate the beginning of World War III." Weekdays, in the hour between the time Doug and Meggan returned from school and Tom and Elizabeth came home from work, Meggan would barricade herself in her bedroom, scream at the top of her lungs, and telephone Doug's friends to tell embarrassing stories about her brother. Doug compensated for the frustration his sister caused by punching holes in the upstairs hallway doors. Said Elizabeth, "We laugh sometimes about putting the house up for sale. We have so much work to do just to fix the stuff that Douglas has broken because he gets so angry."

The situation among Elizabeth, Meggan, and Doug reached a crisis point during the summer between Meggan's sixth and seventh grade. "I literally got into a near-homicidal rage toward Meggan," said Elizabeth. "I not only wanted her out of my life, I wanted her dead." After a series of discussions, the family agreed that Meggan had to go away for a while; separation was the only answer. "We sent her to a working farm in Lake Placid, New York, called North Country School. It's a really neat place."

Interestingly, Meggan seemed more than willing to go off on her own and had once suggested that her parents rent an apartment near her high school and provide her with an allowance until she could find work to support herself. Private school was not her preference, but she quickly adjusted. At the preliminary interview at North Country, Meggan exhibited none of the insecurity and shyness that might normally be expected of an adolescent entering a new peer group. Meggan "walked in like she owned the place. Everyone liked her." They had visited North Country in the autumn. When Meggan returned after Christmas to begin the winter semester, Elizabeth gave her a button which said: "Back By Popular Demand."

As the Scanlons continually discovered, Meggan had never lacked socialization skills, either with peers or adults, who were impressed with her poise and charm—despite Tom's and Elizabeth's attempts to caution innocent bystanders. "At the beginning of every school year, I would wait a couple of weeks and then make special appointments with Meg's teachers. I'd say, 'Let me tell you about my daughter. She may do things that are a little odd. Just tell her exactly what you want her to do and always give her explicit instructions, and she'll probably be okay.' When I told this to her third-grade teacher, the woman jumped down my throat: 'Why don't you be your daughter's friend instead of coming in here and telling lies about her?'

"It happened all the time. At the beginning of every school year, I would attempt to tell the teachers the truth about Meggan, and they would look at me like I was crazy. 'Oh, she just seems so pleasant; I'm sure we're going to have a wonderful year.' At the end of every school year, the teachers were singing a different tune—total relief that they had survived and would probably not have to face Meggan again. Her behaviors were unpredictable and bizarre. She would wander away from class and be found sitting somewhere in a sink. Or, in the middle of a lecture given by one of her teachers, she would start to clean out her desk. Her favorite trick was to disappear during fire drills. The teachers would be so mad because they were required to know where every kid is. She'd come back, but wouldn't be able to tell them where she had gone."

Unless people knew Meggan from day-to-day contact over many months, they refused to believe that she was so difficult and different. Even friends who attempted to empathize with the Scanlons' frustration were overflowing with unrealistic and insensitive advice: "Just throw her out of the house," the Scanlons had been repeatedly told. But how can parents turn their backs on their daughter? Tough love works much better on other people's children.

Finally, Elizabeth and Tom simply refused to discuss their troubles amongst the people with whom they had the most in common. For twelve years, they have been playing pinochle every month with a group of their oldest and dearest friends. "These days, we sit in the car before joining them, hold each other's hands, and pledge we will not talk about our problems, no matter what happens."

When asked if they resented their friends for not being responsive and empathetic, Tom and Elizabeth refer to a very short story written by Emily Perl Kingsley, the mother of a severely handicapped child, called "Holland."

When you are going to have a baby, it is like planning a fabulous vacation trip—to Italy. You buy a bunch of guidebooks and make your wonderful plans. The Coliseum. The Michelangelo *David*. The gondolas in Venice. You may learn some handy phrases in Italian. It's all very exciting.

After months of eager anticipation, the day finally arrives. You pack your bags and off you go. Several hours later, the plane lands. The stewardess comes in and says, "Welcome to Holland."

"Holland?" you say. "What do you mean Holland? I signed up for Italy. I'm supposed to be in Italy. All my life I have dreamed of going to Italy."

But there has been a change in the flight plan. They've landed in Holland and there you must stay.

The important thing is that they haven't taken you to a horrible filthy place, full of pestilence, famine, and disease. It's just a different place.

So you must go out and buy new guidebooks. And you must learn a whole new language. And you will meet a whole new group of people that you would have never met.

It's just a different place. It's slower-paced than Italy, less flashy than Italy. But after you've been there for a while and you catch your breath, you notice that Holland has windmills, Holland has tulips. Holland even has Rembrandts.

But everyone you know is busy coming and going from Italy, and they are all bragging about what a wonderful time they had there. And for the rest of your life, you will say, "That's where I was supposed to go. That's what I had planned."

And the pain will never, ever, ever go away, because the loss of that dream is a very significant loss.

But if you spend your life mourning the fact that you didn't get to Italy, you may never be free to enjoy the very special, the very lovely things about Holland.

The fact that Elizabeth and Tom Scanlon have adopted the story of "Holland" as a metaphor for their life with Meggan is heartwarming, but a denial of reality typical of families with mentally ill kids. Holland was different from Italy, but it became unique enough to be enjoyed. Meggan was special and unique, but fundamentally flawed. Rather than learning to live with Meggan, the Scanlons were beginning to acknowledge that life with Meggan might soon be impossible to endure.

THE SCANLONS ARE not alone, nor is Elizabeth particularly unusual in her anger toward her daughter and her inability to maintain a clear and balanced perspective. I have interviewed dozens of parents whose lives mirror the Scanlons' debilitating desperation, including Beverly M, whom I met at a workshop for parents with ADHD children. When the session began and I introduced myself and explained my project, Beverly, a short, chunky woman with gray-speckled hair, immediately launched into a tirade about how difficult it was for parents who "owned one of these children" to get anyone to understand the hardship under which they lived. "Walk a mile in my shoes before you think you understand how we feel. We'll see how long you last."

Although I thought that Elizabeth Scanlon was more nervous, volatile, and desperate, I felt more sympathy for Beverly. Her son David was only twelve, while Meggan was fifteen, and so the parental struggle of adolescence was just beginning rather than midway. Meggan was bright and obviously independent, whereas David was developmentally delayed. Elizabeth Scanlon was angry, but Beverly was bitter and beaten. She told her story in the matter-of-fact way of a person whose options have been exhausted. Hope has eluded her.

"We got him when he was nine and a half months. He had been left to lie without moving. The foster parents didn't pick him up; they didn't roll him over; they didn't cuddle him or do anything to get him stimulated. We put him in United Cerebral Palsy infant clinic, and within three months they had him up and walking. But he's never really walked. One day, all of a sudden, he took off and ran across the room. He's been running ever since. There have been days when my husband has come home from work and I've just handed him over and said, 'If I don't leave now, we'll have a funeral tomorrow.'

"I have been so angry, so anxious, so upset, so rattled because of this kid. One day I was so discombobulated that I just grabbed him and threw him across the room. He's got a scar today a good inch and a half long. He sometimes asks about that scar, and I explain that that was not the best day in my life. He had hit our new baby, who was bleeding across the eye. And he'd pooped his pants I don't know how many times. He peed on the floor. He'd done just about everything to rattle a mother. I was at my wits' end. I looked at him afterwards and I remember thinking, 'If that isn't child abuse, what is?' It was then that I realized that I needed help, he needed help, my husband needed help, the whole family needed help. It's been very, very difficult."

David's inability to cooperate with the rest of the family—and the "tough love" techniques Beverly has been counseled to enforce—have led to frustrating and embarrassing moments, the most memorable of which was a Sunday morning at church. "Daddy leaves early for leadership meetings; I come along later with the kids. Meetings—we are Mormons—begin at 9:00 A.M. We have to leave by at least a quarter to nine to be on time. But David would always mess around and refuse to dress." One winter morning, she packed him into the car with only his underwear on. "We got in the car, and the car was freezing cold. He complained about how cold he was, and I said, 'You'll have to wait about ten minutes and by that time we'll be at church.'

" 'What will the people say about me at church?'

"I said, 'That's too bad. You should have thought about that when I told you it was time to get dressed. You had forty-five minutes. You didn't do it. Tough.'

"We got there. He picked his way across the parking lot, walked inside. The church leaders looked down their noses at me. We're talking about an extremely conservative group. David knew that he had totally fouled up. Finally he begged his sister to let him wear her coat, which she did. The church leaders told me not to bring him to church in his underwear anymore. But I haven't had any problem with him since. Now I set the timer and say, 'Get ready for church.' He's the first one dressed."

Excerpts from Beverly's diary illustrate the daily pressure of dealing without help with a child with serious mental health problems.

Saturday, March 18, 1989

Cloudy, rain, then snow. Quite cold. David got into the shoe polish while I was gone and got it all over our bed. . . . We all went to Giant Eagle (supermarket). What a disaster!

Monday, April 3

Cloudy. David came home. He's been passing out one dollar bills and asking for money. (I think he's been stealing $.) He's just a sneaky little kid! Always has been.

Saturday, April 15

Clear. Went to the circus. It was the saddest circus I've ever seen . . . only one clown. David carried on terribly through the entire second act, because five of the kids were going to be a part of the circus. . . . I couldn't let him go because he's so unpredictable.

Sunday, July 16

. . . David messed up in his Sunday school class and got put out of the room left to his own devices. He . . . pitched stones at passing cars. He connected with one and put a very small dent in the roof. The guy was steamed. . . . Sent him to bed at 7:00 P.M.

August 6

Cloudy, some rain. Took the kids to the park. David pooped his pants. Margaret brought him home (he waddled like a duck or an eighty-nine-year-old man) and cleaned him up.

August 7

Only 62 degrees today. David came home with a negative. He looked so pathetic—he said, "Mommy, I really tried." My heart went out to him. . . .

August 30

Clear. So——I was stuck *again with* the kids. There's no break from this endless drudge.

November 12

Clear. David spent the afternoon pulling toys apart with screwdrivers. Now he has a lot of broken toys. My head ached really bad.

Tuesday, January 16, 1990

Cloudy. Got a call about 8:15 P.M. Seems like David learned the emergency phone number for ambulance, fire, police . . . so he got on the phone and called them. What a ruckus he raised. Now he has a record at the police. He should have been arrested, they said, and put into detention for what he did. Why me?

2

THE CONCEPT OF a predisposed temperament in children ("temperamentally difficult" was the diagnosis the Scanlons had accepted for Meggan) has been frequently debated. It contradicts the long-held belief, initially proposed by the seventeenth-century philosopher John Locke, that a newborn child's mind is a *tabula rasa* or blank slate on which the adult world may write or create character, morality, and knowledge.

Leading proponents of the existence of temperament in newborns were psychiatrists Alexander Thomas and Stella Chess, who in the late 1960s and early 1970s conducted a study of 141 toddler-age children in seventy-five families that divided the majority of children into three temperamental categories. On one extreme, 40 percent of the children in their sample were "easy," characterized by pleasant mood, regularity in body functions, and a positive approach to new situations. On the other end of the spectrum were "difficult children," those displaying irregular body functions, sleeping, and feeding; intense moods; inability to adapt to environment. Ten percent of the Thomas and Chess sample fell into this category, which is where Meggan Scanlon would be placed.

Following their subjects over a period of years, Thomas and Chess discovered that seven out of ten "difficult" children eventually developed behavioral problems that called for psychiatric intervention, compared to about one in five "easy" children—statistics that generate just as many questions as answers. If there exists a predisposed temperament within a child from birth, then why did a significant minority of easy children show evidence of behavioral problems while an even more significant minority of the difficult children did not? The basic question of the existence of temperament is only one example of the differences between the hard sciences, where only facts prevail, and the behavioral sciences, where facts are often contradicted by an ever-changing and puzzling reality.

The medical world has made such incredible strides over the past quarter century, with magnetic resonance imaging (MRI) providing amazing insight into human anatomy and heretofore unimaginable surgical accomplishments such as open-heart surgery and fetal transplantation, that it is difficult to truly understand and accept the very primitive state of psychiatry. Psychiatrists are basically blind as to how the brain and the mind work—or even the subtle differences between the two.

Although a myriad of medications, talk therapies, and behavioral modification programs have sometimes been successful in changing patterns of behavior, it is often a hit-and-miss proposition. Nothing can be taken for granted. The brain is a "mysterious black box," a psychiatrist once told me. "We can't see what's in there, but we know there are a lot of chemicals, and they are doing something weird because there are a bunch of strange symptoms showing up in our patients. So we open the lid, throw some drugs in, have some conversations with patients about their feelings, and sometimes the symptoms get better." And sometimes the symptoms don't, he said. And sometimes you learn after years of trying to help the patient that you have been treating him for the wrong problems.

Up until very recently, almost all research into mental illness has been done on adult patients, with the assumption that viable treatments would eventually filter down into the pediatric population. What has been discovered, however, is that children cannot be uniformly diagnosed and treated based upon experience garnered from work with adults. Children who are depressed, for example, are often oppositional and irritable, whereas adults usually sink into an abyss of quiet despair.

Medications that have been effective in treating some adults often have little impact upon kids. Studies have shown that children may respond to antidepressant medication no better than they respond to similar regimens of placebos. Unlike adults, the child is an ever-changing commodity; puberty will often cause emotional stress that complicates the diagnosis and treatment of mental illness.

Significantly, Thomas and Chess do not focus solely on the biological or genetic roots of temperament, rejecting the classic "nature-nurture" debate as too arbitrary and choosing a "constitutionalist" approach in which personality is shaped by the constant interplay of temperament and environment. Freud pointed out that neuroses are only acquired through early childhood, while John Watson, the father of behaviorist thinking, often in theoretical conflict with Freudian psychodynamic principles, often observed that a child's character can easily be spoiled by bad handling. Perhaps the damage can never be repaired.

As an overall blanket term for the interaction of biology and environment, Thomas and Chess have developed what they call the concept of "goodness of fit," which results when the demands and expectations of the environment are consonant with the individual's capacities and characteristics. "When this is so, healthy psychological development and functioning is likely. 'Poorness of fit,' on the other hand, results when the individual does not have the capacities or characteristics to cope adequately with the environmental demands and expectations. Excessive stress is then likely to occur, and the child or adult becomes at high risk for behavior problem development."

As I followed the Scanlons through the heartache of therapy and beyond, I thought often of the "goodness of fit" and "poorness of fit" concepts proposed by Alexander Thomas and Stella Chess. Did Meggan Scanlon suffer from serious psychiatric problems from birth? Or were the temperamental styles of Tom and Elizabeth simply incompatible with their daughter's personality—or both? Could anything have been done by the Scanlons or their doctors to have shielded the family from such constant torment? Or had the Scanlons been doomed from the very beginning?

There are no definitive answers to these questions—only a series of indications and possibilities which may well be accurate, or, conversely, could also be contradictory and misleading. The muddy concept of a genetic linkage in psychiatric illness is an ideal example of the scientific confusion illustrated by Tom, Elizabeth, and Meggan Scanlon.

"Tom and Elizabeth come from strange families," Debbie Rubin told me as she leafed through the careful history she had taken at the time of Meggan's admission. "Tom's aunt has had many hospitalizations and was treated with ECT [electroconvulsive or "shock" therapy]. A relative committed suicide and a nephew is learning-disabled. Elizabeth has a history of depression and a record of physical complaints that are probably very real to her that I suspect have to do with stress."

Elizabeth added familial details. "My grandfather was a terrible, violent, demented man. My mother can't talk about him at all. She's seventy-two years old and the mention of her father just brings her to tears." As a child, Elizabeth's brother was extraordinarily aggressive. "He would do anything to pick a fight. To this day, rather than say hello, he'll punch you in the arm."

On the other hand, Elizabeth wonders what her history really means. "It's so easy for people to say, 'It was your mother who did this to you—or your father or your brother.' " If her mother can be blamed for Elizabeth's own feelings of inadequacy and depression, then how much can she be blamed for Meggan's problems? "Maybe it has been my fault. What did I do wrong?" she asks. "I must have done something wrong."

Genetic linkage does not explain all or perhaps even most of the reasons for mental illness. Depression is a prime example. Medications for unrelated diseases could cause depression in some patients. Four of ten women who take birth control pills suffer from depression. Even medications originally intended to help emotionally disturbed children can trigger a depressive episode in some patients.

Janice Egeland of the University of Miami and her colleagues performed a genetic analysis of an inherited form of manic depression in an Amish family. Because of their large family size, detailed genealogical records, and genetic isolation, the Amish are ideal for such undertakings. The 15,000 U.S. members of this religious sect have all descended from thirty couples who migrated to America in the early nineteenth century. Egeland was unable to identify the exact gene, but she localized it on the short arm of chromosome 11 so that geneticist John Kelsoe of the National Institute of Mental Health could have an excellent chance of finding it. Instead, Kelsoe discovered that he could not duplicate Egeland's work. Egeland had done nothing wrong, but the search was becoming more complicated. Egeland and Kelsoe speculated that there are perhaps two or more genes for manic depression, one of which may be on chromosome 11—but may not.

A similar scenario was played out in the pages of the *Journal of the American Medical Association* (JAMA) concerning a genetic link that predisposed some people to alcoholism. In an article in April 1990, researchers at the University of Texas reported that a gene existed in 69 percent of their sampling of alcoholics, versus in only 20 percent of their control subjects. In a follow-up study conducted by the National Institute of Alcohol Abuse and Alcoholism, and published the following January in JAMA, no significant difference in the number of alcoholics and nonalcoholics who carried the same gene was indicated, thus demonstrating the continued difficulty in pinpointing cause and cure in mental illness. Recent studies have confirmed the role of heredity in IQ, hyperactivity, schizophrenia, autism, and aggression, but it remains to be seen if such work will be more specifically duplicated and confirmed.

Even if it becomes possible to show that specific mental illnesses run in families, it doesn't necessarily guarantee actualization. Stress during pregnancy, for example, drugs, malnutrition, even cigarette smoking, may cause undue harm. Lead poisoning from paint or trauma suffered in an automobile accident may also trigger a biological dysfunction in the brain.

The question has been debated for the past century. It is a confrontation of extremes: chemistry versus free will; nature or nurture; heredity versus environment; fate as opposed to responsibility. The truth undoubtedly falls somewhere in the middle. Freud was right. Watson was wrong. Or Freud was wrong and Watson was right. Part of the brain is hard-wired in advance of birth and part of the brain, like clay, is malleable through experience. As Daniel E. Koshland, editor of *Science*, explains: "Some individuals who have normal genes become overwhelmed by adversity in their environment, sink into depression, and attempt suicide. At the other extreme, some who have loving parents, ideal schooling, and a stress-free life are overwhelmed by their internal chemistry and also succumb to depression and suicidal intentions. Still others are pushed into depression by stresses that are easily surmounted by individuals with different genetic components. . . . Our judges, journalists, legislators, and philosophers have been slow to learn this lesson."

3

I WAS APPREHENSIVE the first time I entered Western Psych, uncomfortable that someone might see me walking into a mental hospital—and think that maybe I belonged there. This is not an enlightened point of view, but it is representative. With the exception of AIDS, there is perhaps no greater negative public stigma than that of mental illness. In 1972, Senator Thomas Eagleton was forced to withdraw as the Democratic vice-presidential nominee because of public reaction against previous ECT treatment. His liberal running mate, Senator George McGovern, requested Eagleton's resignation. Eighteen years later, in the Florida gubernatorial election, former Senator Lawton Chiles was attacked by his opponent for having been treated for depression. The American Psychiatric Association (APA) supported Chiles, who eventually was elected, but studies conducted by the National Institute of Mental Health (NIMH) demonstrate that "many health-care professionals harbor unconscious, unstated negative feelings about their mental patients."

On a societal level, ex-convicts are more acceptable than former mental patients, according to NIMH. Asked to rank twenty-one categories of disabilities from the least offensive to the most, respondents placed mental illness at the bottom of the list. Victims who have been burdened by both mental illness and cancer report that mental illness caused greater pain, in part because of the obstacles presented by society during recovery. According to the Child Mental Health Interest Group of the National Mental Health Association (NMHA), the younger the mentally ill child, the worse the impact of stigma is on both parents and child: They feel more shame.

, Because of such stigma, many parents have secretly confided that they sometimes wish their child were retarded rather than mentally ill. Not only do retarded children receive more services, but families are accorded much more public support. "Parents of mentally retarded children are not blamed for the child's retardation," says Lynn Alms of United Mental Health, Inc., the leading advocacy group in western Pennsylvania, who directs a support group attended by the Scanlons. "Parents may feel guilt about genetic problems, but such disorders are not caused by poor parenting. It's an act of God. With mentally ill kids, the parents are constantly questioned and doubted." The concept of the "refrigerator mother" causing autism has only recently been discredited.

Although this stigma is an age-old problem, the modern media is partially to blame for the prevalence of this attitude. Newspapers stress a history of mental disorder in the backgrounds of people who commit crimes, while in many TV dramas mentally ill people are portrayed as perpetrators of violent and diabolic acts. But NIMH studies have demonstrated that only 2 percent of former mental patients pose any danger to society, compared to drunk drivers—for whom Americans display an astonishing tolerance—who are directly responsible for half of all automobile fatalities. Because they are basically physically healthy, mentally ill adults and children, if rehabilitated, are an untapped source and sorely needed force of intelligence and energy, with an excellent potential of helping to elevate our nation from decay and malaise. The children I met at Western Psych and at many group homes are very sick, but the vast majority could be helped if government and society would provide resources and understanding. Instead, we have created a downward spiral of failure and defeat that will impact upon our society for generations.

In a 1990 study, published in the *Journal of the American Academy of Child and Adolescent Psychiatry* (AACAP), psychiatrist Sarah Fox, of Columbia University College of Physicians and Surgeons, showed that of fifty parent-child pairs from homeless families housed in New York City hotels the great majority of homeless children four to ten years old were functioning at far below the average cognitive level for children their same age. One third of the children were not attending school and one third had repeated a grade; 40 percent of the children were reported by their parents to have significant emotional and behavioral problems; and 75 percent of the children were found to have moderate to severe impairment on the Children's Global Assessment Scale, a behavior-oriented measurement. Approximately one third of the parents were depressed, and approximately one third gave a history of emotional problems.

According to Dr. Thomas Oliver, president of the American Board of Pediatrics, our child health care system requires a total reprioritization. Child poverty in the U.S. could be completely eliminated with an influx of $17 billion—only one fourth of 1 percent of our gross national product. "In America today we spend $22 billion a year on alcohol, and $52 billion on new cars, annually," states Dr. Oliver. A pediatrician will charge approximately $35 for a well-baby checkup, which is close to cost, while the government through Medicaid will only provide $15, thus discouraging participation of both parents and doctors. Similarly, most community health centers provide reduced fees for therapy and/or counseling—perhaps $18 for a 45-minute hour. "This is a bargain basement rate for wealthy people or those with reasonable insurance coverage, but $18 is completely out of reach for the homeless and disenfranchised."

Approximately 16 million children and adolescents completely lack health-care coverage, an increase of 14 percent over the past decade. America, the world's remaining superpower, is currently 22nd in infant mortality rate and 26th in the percentage of low birth-weight babies—behind countries as poor as Bulgaria. Low birth-weight babies are generally born with a normal IQ, but have a much higher risk of developing learning problems. In fact, 12 percent of U.S. children actually start school with generally preventable learning problems, including lead poisoning, untreated ear infections, malnutrition, and prenatal exposure to drugs.

Ironically and unfortunately, reports, discussions, and exposés about lack of adequate treatment for children with mental health problems compose an old and tired melody. As far back as 1909, a White House conference on children stressed the need for new programs to care for mentally disturbed children. Twenty-one years later at a subsequent White House conference, participants pointedly stated that mentally ill children deserved the right to develop as all other children. In a 1969 report entitled "Crisis in Child Mental Health," the Joint Commission on Mental Health of Children illustrated how a large proportion of children and adolescents with mental disorders received either no care whatsoever or inappropriate and often unnecessarily restrictive care under questionable conditions in state mental hospitals. In 1978, the President's Commission on Mental Health repeated the Joint Commission's findings, stressing that the only substantive changes that had occurred in the preceding decade had been for the worse.

In perhaps the most prestigious and widely quoted study, *Unclaimed Children*, supported and published in book form in 1982 by the Children's Defense Fund, author Jane Knitzer estimates that two thirds of the seriously disturbed children in the U.S. are not receiving the services they need, while countless others are inappropriately served. Most recently, in its 1989 report, *Research on Children and Adolescents with Mental, Behavioral and Developmental Disorders*, the Institute of Medicine (IOM) maintained that less than 25 percent of the children in the U.S. suffering from mental illness receive any treatment whatsoever. It isn't a question of nothing changing, as much as it is a situation that is rapidly worsening, Knitzer recently told me. Eighty percent of the physically handicapped children in this country are adequately served, yet for serious emotional disturbance, the evidence is that less than 30 percent are, even when they are noticed.

The situation is even worse for minority children, according to a recent Child Welfare League of America colloquium: "If you are an adolescent and black and you are seriously emotionally disturbed, the chances are that you will end up in the justice system, rather than in a treatment setting. If you are a Native American child and you are seriously emotionally disturbed, you will likely go without treatment, or be removed legally and geographically from your family and tribe. If you are a child who is Hispanic and seriously emotionally disturbed, the assessment is not going to be in your own language. If you are an Asian child and seriously emotionally disturbed, you will probably never come to the attention of the health-care system."

In its study, the IOM concluded that there are very few child psychiatrists in the United States able to sustain a major research commitment. "Fewer than 100 academic child psychiatrists are currently devoting 30 percent or more of their time to research; fewer than 20 can be considered full-time investigators. In the area of social work, fewer than 300 doctoral degrees are awarded annually and only a small fraction on topics related to childhood mental disorders." In 1988, NIMH spent $2.1 million for research training related to children and adolescents—approximately the same amount of money it cost to purchase one M-1A1 Abrams tank used in the Persian Gulf War, of which the Pentagon currently owns 8,000. Conservatively, the IOM suggested that the annual budget for research training should be nearly $20 million—equal to the cost of only ten M-1A1 tanks.

Politicians fail to understand the cost-effectiveness of scientific research. Approximately $70 million was expended for research and prevention measures in the development of the Sabin polio vaccine—including funds put toward Jonas Salk's Nobel Prize–winning work. According to Dr. Oliver, "It is estimated that if the Sabin vaccine had not been discovered until 1989, $40 billion would have been spent in the care, treatment, and rehabilitation of children and adults contracting polio." Even accounting for inflation, the spiraling expenses of mental illness make the investment in polio research and the subsequent savings seem minuscule. Over the first six months of 1992, for example, 19 percent of the adult U.S. population will suffer a diagnosable mental disorder—at a cost of approximately $250 billion annually. There are no similar up-to-date predictions about expenditures for children with mental health problems, but the National Prevention Coalition of the NMHA has estimated that the cost of direct care, combined with social-welfare programs and lost productivity, in 1981 was $54 billion.

4

THE NORTH COUNTRY SCHOOL in Lake Placid, New York, had seemed ideal for Meggan Scanlon, a place where she could have structure, supervision, and supervisory patience on a twenty-four-hour basis. A dozen or so students live in a large farmhouse, with houseparents constantly accountable for their whereabouts. Meggan could participate in a wide variety of winter sports, while caring for a barnful of animals and enjoying regular horseback riding. The setting was idyllic— perhaps a little too idyllic for Meggan, one year older and considerably more sexually mature than most of the other students.

At first, her experience at North Country from January 1990 through the spring semester was quite positive. In such a structured and stimulating outdoor atmosphere, Meggan both mellowed and matured, learning for the first time how to exert a measure of self-control, while scoring high marks academically. Totally enjoying their quiet respite from a lifetime of household turmoil, Elizabeth, Tom, and Doug were healed and rested when Meggan returned home for the summer, fortified with a more positive attitude. No one will know whether the Scanlons had actually discovered a workable compromise with Meggan at North

Country because circumstances beyond everyone's control began to lead the family toward imminent disaster.

Because of a previous bicycle accident in which she broke her jaw, Meggan was scheduled for reconstructive surgery that summer. The Scanlons had known that sooner or later surgery would be necessary, but had hoped to delay the inevitable until Meggan was more psychologically prepared. Now it could not be put off any longer. Afterwards, her jaw was wired shut, thus forcing her to sustain herself on liquids. Abstinence from solid food combined with the heat of the summer would have caused emotional trauma for any adult, let alone a "temperamentally difficult" teenager. To make matters worse, Meggan fell and broke her heel and was put into a non-weight-bearing cast. Without solid food or the benefit of exercise, Meggan's frustration accelerated. The fragile peace in effect since Meggan's return from North Country was quickly shattered. Meggan's cast was not removed until the day before she was scheduled to return to North Country in the fall. Doug, Elizabeth, and Tom were emotionally spent. "We were exhilarated to say good-bye," said Tom. "Even if we had been told that we could never see her again, we would have been happy to let her go."

At North Country, Meggan was excused from physical education during her recuperation, yet in her thoughtless and whimsical way, she would suddenly run across the campus or climb out of her window in the middle of the night to rendezvous with a boyfriend. Seeing that she was physically active, her counselors required her to participate in organized hiking, swimming, and horseback riding, despite her objections. Every night, Meggan phoned her parents, hysterically claiming she was being physically abused. The Scanlons eventually convinced school administrators to allow Meggan a certain leeway because of her stressful summer, hoping that she could work back into the rhythm of the North Country experience. As a result, she was faced with significant blocks of free time. For some people they would be considered a great luxury; for Meggan, they were a prescription for disaster.

Walking in the woods one afternoon, Meggan came upon a cabin, abandoned during the school year but used in the summer by art students. For reasons she has never been able to explain, Meggan suddenly snapped, breaking into the cabin, splattering paint all over the walls, smashing windows, shredding screens, and pounding nails into the floor. When her tantrum ended, she filled a large plastic trash bag full of art supplies and hid it in the woods nearby. She then led her teachers back to the trash bag, claiming she had stumbled across it and that she had heard a great commotion coming from inside the cabin. Minutes later, the destruction was discovered.

At first, Meggan insisted she had had nothing to do with the ransacking, even though the evidence pointed to her. "She'd call us on the phone and say, 'They're blaming me; I didn't do it,' " Tom said. "I'd say, 'Well, Meggan, the truth will eventually come out.' " Three weeks later, Meggan confessed and was suspended from North Country.

Elizabeth remembers seeing Meggan for the first time when she returned home after the suspension. Her eyes were shiny with tears and she was incredibly frightened, not by what she had done to the cabin, but by the anger exploding inside of her that had led to the destructive act. Meggan could not actually remember raging through that cabin, but she could remember stopping, breathless, suddenly standing in the middle of the cabin and seeing for the first time the destruction she had caused. And she could remember hearing a bell, reminding her that she was expected back at the school for classes. She had no memory of doing anything—only the retrospective knowledge that she was wholly responsible for what had been done.

They were in Dr. Cohen's office the following morning, with Tom and Elizabeth insisting for what seemed like the hundredth time that the opinion that nothing could be done about Meggan's "temperament" was not an adequate answer. "There is a psychiatric diagnosis here," Elizabeth insisted. "There must be a way to treat it."

But Elizabeth felt that Dr. Cohen considered the incident at North Country a response to Meggan's anger after being pent up over the entire summer. She had exploded. When Meggan's suspension ended, she returned to North Country a few weeks later and was permitted to take walks to vent her anger or go into the bathroom and scream. Meggan was obligated to clean up the mess she had made at the cabin, and she worked hard. She was contrite and promised she would never do anything like that again. But Elizabeth and Tom knew their daughter had lost a significant measure of her very fragile control. They braced themselves for the worst.

"The houseparents lived downstairs, with all the kids upstairs, sharing bedrooms and bathrooms," Tom explained. "We had expressed concern about the closeness of the boys and girls, but the possibility of anything going on was pretty much discounted—it was supposed to be a very brotherly-sisterly situation." Not for Meggan, especially in her desperate state of mind. By midsemester, Meggan became involved in a "sexual situation" with a couple of boys who lived in her house and was once again suspended from the school. This time she would not return.

Assuming that Meggan would be away from home in the fall, Tom and Elizabeth had scheduled a vacation/business trip to San Francisco. Because Meggan and Doug had to be watched so closely, the Scanlons had not taken a vacation alone in many years, and they were determined to go through with this one, despite the dangers. "Meggan stayed with Tom's parents. I don't know what planet I was on when I agreed to that, but I must have been out of my mind," Elizabeth said.

"Meggan went on a shopping binge. We never buy clothes in stores. We buy our clothes in resale shops, and for us to go to a mall and spend money—hundreds of dollars—on clothing is just completely unlike Meggan. She likes resale shops, thinks the stuff is great. For her to spend all this money . . . and not be able to explain why, was baffling. Then she got into an argument with my in-laws over what windows were to be opened in the house—and ran away. My sister-in-law and my mother-in-law were both terrified." This incident had been a shock to people who insisted that Meggan was perfectly normal.

"Once again, when we returned home, we took her to see Dr. Cohen. Looking back, I sometimes get mad, wasting a lot of time and energy, because we must have asked him, I don't know how many dozens of times, if we should be putting Meggan into Western Psych or some other hospital. But he continued to insist that Meggan had a personality [temperament] disorder, and that there wasn't anything anybody could do to confirm or deny the diagnosis.

"I would say, 'Is she mentally ill? Is this a treatable illness?' And I was told repeatedly, 'No, it's not.'

" 'Is there someplace she should go? Is there anyplace in the world that she belongs where she could be helped—because she is not being helped at home.' If Dr. Cohen had told me to put her in group therapy in Chicago, I would have done it. But the feeling was that the best environment was at home with the two of us who cared for her—which was pretty much how it had been before North Country and through the winter and spring since her return."

Then an acquaintance from their support group suggested Meggan might have a sleep disorder, based upon her oppositional behavior at night, and recommended an evaluation at the Western Psych sleep lab. They made an appointment with its director, pediatrician Ronald Dahl. "Half an hour into the interview, he split us up and interviewed us alone," said Tom. "Later he told me that he thought she was bipolar, meaning manic depressive. You could have knocked me over with a feather. I said, 'Why do you think that?' He said, 'Well, observing her, listening to what you have both told me, it's classic. It is a textbook case.' "

TWENTY MILLION— one in twelve—Americans suffer from depressive illness; one in ten of those are estimated to have bipolar disorder, a condition identified by periods of severe depression interspersed with episodes of uncontrollable elation, restlessness, racing thoughts, and delusions of grandeur.

To learn more about bipolar illness, I watched a video at the Western Psych library entitled *Four Lives: A Portrait of Manic Depression* (another term for bipolar illness). The video began by explaining that the moods of manic-depressives "swerve erratically and often unaccountably. At times, victims feel excessive energy and elation. They may become involved in outlandish and grandiose schemes. At other times, they feel an all-consuming misery—weeks and months pass and they are barely able to function or even think normally. This disorder can ravage families and devastate lives. It can be fatal. One in six afflicted with manic depression commits suicide."

Watching the production, I was struck by how much the symptoms and ramifications of bipolar disease mirrored Meggan's behaviors. In the video, Houston psychiatrist Michael Schlesser explained that mania is often very one-sided. Individuals cannot sit down and engage another person in a meaningful conversation; they cannot listen. They only pick up parts of the conversation, being distracted by a painting on the wall, or a car going by, or a thought they suddenly had. They also have an urge to talk. They will speak rapidly although the speech doesn't keep up with their thinking, and they will go from one subject to another without meaningful and obvious connection. Their moods rapidly alternate from a manic state to a depressed state. "Patients with mood disorders—in particular, manic-depressives—very likely will have delusions and hallucinations," said Schlesser.

The video also featured an interview with the husband of a patient, Joanne, who explained that when his wife was in her manic phases she wanted to have sex every day. She would take the kids to school and come back and want him to leave work, get into bed, and make love. She would also call people she hadn't seen in fifteen or twenty years and go on wild shopping sprees. Another woman, the wife of a manic-depressive, reminded me of Elizabeth Scanlon talking about Meggan. "He goes from being a considerate, kind, fun, real, neat person to being an egomaniac," she said of her husband. "He's always right, totally perfect, and he's omnipotent. He knows everything. He's done everything. He's been everywhere. When he talks to you it's like a knife going through your heart."

Many creative and driven people have been known to be bipolar, including writer Virginia Woolf, photographer Diane Arbus, and artist Vincent van Gogh, as well as Alexander the Great and Winston Churchill, who called the disease from which he suffered "the black dog." George Frideric Handel composed the *Messiah*, which requires four hours to perform, in three weeks during an extended manic episode. After one of his frequent hospitalizations, Broadway director Joshua Logan asked: "How can I go back to the theater after all the galloping whispers and all of the people who have seen me in this strange state?" The poet Robert Lowell, in his poem "Since 1939," wrote of manic-depressives: "if we see a light at the end of the tunnel / it's the light of an oncoming train."

DR. DAHL ARRANGED an appointment for the Scanlons with a colleague, Scott Waterman, at Western Psych's Affective Disorders outpatient clinic. "Meggan was interviewed for maybe thirty seconds before they decided to admit her to the hospital. We spent the entire day there, taking a battery of tests, until there was no doubt in anyone's mind." Meggan finally had a diagnosis. There was actually something specific, scientific, and psychiatric wrong with her—a reason for her behavior—after all of these years. Meggan was a manic-depressive. "It sounds perverse," Tom said, "but we were overjoyed."

DANIEL

INVOLVEMENT WITH DANIEL as his "big brother"—or "mentor"
as it is more fashionably called today—triggered my interest in investi-
gating the lack of options facing kids with mental health problems. The
parents of some of the kids at the group home where I first met Daniel
were either in jail or had been declared temporarily unfit to care for their
children. A few, like Daniel, had no active familial connections at all.

Daniel was short and slender when I met him, with very serious pale
blue eyes, curly dark hair, and a little ponytail. What struck me about
Daniel was how delicate he was—and clean. He showered four times a
day. In contrast to the other kids' rooms, Daniel's clothes were neatly
folded and his bed had sheets made with hospital corners. You could
bounce a penny off Daniel's sheets, just like in the military. Little
paintings and drawings decorated Daniel's wall—stick figures, houses,
and automobiles fashioned in crude squares and straight lines. This was
not skillful work for a ten-year-old, let alone a child nearing thirteen.

When the conversation became strained and awkward during our
first few meetings, Daniel would open a battered notebook, take out
sheets of lined loose-leaf paper and begin to carefully recopy three essays
he had recently completed. I peeked over his shoulder as he worked.
Daniel's handwriting was unsteady but very clear, although he had no

sense of punctuation; he would run words together, skipping every other line so that everything he wrote was meticulously neat, like his room. Each time he wrote a word that didn't seem perfect, he would erase it and do it again—or start a new sheet of paper. The essays were very factual, defining three subjects: God, the devil, and plutonium. I later discovered they were copied verbatim out of a ragged, outdated *World Book Encyclopedia* hidden under his bed.

When I had been first briefed about Daniel by the agency that connected us, I was told that he had a great interest in books—and an insatiable curiosity about science and engineering. In fact, when I asked him where he wanted to go first, he selected the library.

Daniel had great plans for the wealth of knowledge he was going to unearth from books—information to guide him toward fulfilling his dream: to build a computer-controlled robot and a bulletproof car, inspired by his favorite television show, "Knight Rider." As soon as he turned eighteen, he planned to change his name to Michael Knight, and then join the police force as a special undercover officer. He told me he had already put his plan into motion. The design for his robot had been drawn; parts were being stored in his locker. I soon came to realize much of this was untrue. Daniel had collected some parts, wires, screws, and so on, none of which would be appropriate for a robot. But more important, he had no concept of what a plan or a design was—only that it was needed. These were ideas and words he had gathered from television and conversations with his counselors without the necessary comprehension to go along with them.

After securing his library card, we wandered aimlessly through the stacks in the children's section until I spotted on a shelf of fiction *The Book of Daniel* by E. L. Doctorow. I slipped it out of the shelf and held it up for him. "Do you see what this is, Daniel?"

He looked at it, nodded, and replied, "Yes, I do." But his eyes were mysteriously dull; there was no spark of recognition.

I began taking other books off the shelves, showing him titles written by men named Daniel. "Do you see this? What does it say?" I asked, and soon realized Daniel could hardly read his own name.

I learned subsequently that his parents had not required him to attend school. When he was first hospitalized with a confusing multiple choice of diagnoses, including schizophrenia, major depression, and post—traumatic stress disorder (PTSD), he was so heavily medicated that studying and learning were nearly impossible. Schizophrenia may no longer be an active diagnosis, but his doctor is certain his depression has been triggered by PTSD, which is similar to shell shock or battle fatigue. Psychiatrists estimate that as many as 800,000 of the 3.5 million men and women who served in the Vietnam War have been affected by PTSD, while children will suffer PTSD after rape, abuse, even birth trauma. Nightmares, sleepwalking, sudden flashbacks—all symptoms of PTSD—constantly plagued Daniel. With no warning, perhaps triggered by a sad TV show or a random memory fragment, Daniel would begin to cry, reliving a painful onslaught of emotion from the past.

Daniel began regularly taking classes only when he moved to the group home two years ago, so his 2.1 grade reading level was understandable in that context. Later, I realized that elementary school reading skills may be the highest level of achievement possible for him.

I had been cautioned about Daniel's robot fixation and obsession with asking questions endlessly, but I was quite unprepared for how little Daniel knew about life—or could do on his own. Just because he had trouble reading and talking—he could not pronounce or understand many words—did not negate his ability to think logically, I had assumed.

As I continued to visit him, the extent of the gaps in his knowledge about the outside world became increasingly apparent. The adults at the group home where he lived or at the special school he attended hardly ever talked with him about subjects other than television and fast food, about which he was satisfactorily knowledgeable, although he was so inundated by TV that he could not distinguish between the story programs and the news. He believed that all hamburgers were made by McDonald's. Every conversation I had with him in the early days became endlessly convoluted because no matter what he asked, I had to backtrack to the absolute beginning in order to put my answer into perspective.

I once told him I was going out of town, flying. He said he had never been in an airplane. "How long does it take to fly on an airplane?"

"It depends upon where you want to go." He nodded as usual, but there was no comprehension in his eyes.

"Well, I am going to New York. You know about New York? Grand

Central station? Times Square?" Another nod, but no recognition. He had never heard of New York.

"How much does it cost to ride in an airplane?" he said.

"Well, where would you like to go?" He looked at me blankly. "Would you like to go to California?" He just looked at me.

"Dan, do you know about the oceans?"

"What's 'oceans'?"

"You know that there are two oceans on either side of our country. Do you know what those oceans are?"

"No."

"The Atlantic and the Pacific. If you fly to California, you'll be at the Pacific Ocean, and if you fly to Florida, you'll be on the Atlantic Ocean."

"How much does it cost to go to Florida?"

"If you go one-way, it will cost you one price, but if you go round-trip you get a discount."

"What's 'round-trip'?"

"It's when you go both ways."

"Well," said Daniel, "what's 'discount'?"

God was a constant topic of conversation. Daniel kept saying, "I don't believe in God because I can't see Him. If God was real, then terrible things wouldn't happen to people. Who made the earth, who made the roads? People say that's God. Where is God? Why can't I see who He is?" The woman who came to the home every Sunday morning to lead religious services told Daniel that he would go to hell if he didn't believe in God.

"Why can't people be nice to one another?" he asked me often. "Why is there prejudice in the world? Why do white people hate black people? Why do some people think Jewish people are ugly? I think I'll become Jewish," he said. "I don't have any other religion."

Daniel eventually discovered that he was born a Catholic, but up until six months before, his caseworkers had never taken the time to search his records to determine his religion.

The resident manager of the group home would not reveal much to me about Daniel's background. It was up to Daniel to tell me what he thought I needed to know—information which he provided in dramatic

44

bits and pieces over the first months of our friendship, usually triggered by a problem he was wrestling with, something pressing on his mind.

"Can I ask you a question?" Almost every conversation began in this way. A question to permit a question.

"Don't you always?" I joked.

"When I was a little kid I was raped by a man. Does that mean I'm gay?"

First we discussed what it meant to be gay. Then we discussed what it meant to be raped. He understood perfectly well; Daniel might not know much about geography, but he was an expert on perversions such as rape. (He could also tell you, step-by-step, how to hot-wire a car, a legacy from an older brother.) I explained that the fact that he had been raped had nothing to do with sexual preferences and nothing to do with him. The person who had raped him was obviously evil or crazy, or both. "Who did that to you?"

A man who lived in the woods outside of his building had sneaked into the apartment one day and raped him. Months later, I learned that Daniel's story might have been distorted; this rapist may have been Daniel's older brother. The entire incident may also have been a figment of Daniel's vivid imagination—which always presented a problem in dealing with Daniel, distinguishing among truth, hallucination, and manipulation.

That day, Daniel was visiting my house for the first time. He sat on a stool at the kitchen counter while I made him his favorite lunch (not counting Pizza Hut pizza): soup and peanut butter and jelly sandwiches on toast, four of them, one after another.

"Can I tell you something?" he said suddenly.

"Sure," I said.

"Nobody in my whole life has ever been nicer to me than you."

I thanked him politely and then went through the rest of our day feeling both an eerie sadness and a warm and appreciative glow. On the one hand, I felt good to be able to give so much to someone, while on the other, it was sad to realize that I was actually doing so very little—giving some attention, being kind, showing some interest.

As the months passed and I invested an increasing amount of time and effort in Daniel, I began to believe that his problems were fixable, that he needed love, attention, discipline, and education, that his disturbances were not as serious as they seemed. Eventually, I came to realize how wrong I was. He did need love, attention, and a real place to belong where there were people he trusted. He also needed a highly structured atmosphere with careful supervision, for he often said and did things of which he was unaware. In addition, I discovered that Daniel's learning disabilities had been complicated by a severe head injury in a fire when he was nine and still living at home.

What does it mean to suffer from learning disabilities? Like Daniel, learning-disabled children have distorted or inadequate auditory and/or visual perception. Dr. Larry B. Silver, clinical professor of psychiatry and associate director of child and adolescent psychiatry at Georgetown University School of Medicine, speaks frequently about the "invisible handicaps" of learning-disabled kids. "They will confuse letters like Bs and Ds and Ps and Qs. They may have trouble figuring out different shapes and positions when they draw designs. They will sit there reading and their eyes will jump words, skip lines, read the same line twice. They will sit at the dinner table, reach for a drink, and knock their glass over because they misjudged the distance. Some children also confuse subtle differences in sound. There are forty-three units of sound in the English alphabet. And they might confuse them, so that words like *blue* and *blow*, or *gnaw* and *no*, or *can* and *can't*, get confused."

I once dedicated an afternoon with Daniel to explaining the difference between *curve* and *curb* and *pier* and *pear*. He simply could not hear the difference and was frequently embarrassed when I attempted to help him. The concepts of "peering" into the distance or "curbing" his appetite completely confounded him.

In its 1991 report, *Beyond Rhetoric*, the National Commission on Children, chaired by West Virginia Senator John D. Rockefeller IV, stated that one in five children between the ages of three and seventeen has a developmental delay, learning disability, or behavioral problem during childhood. "Children with learning disabilities are sometimes thought to be slow learners or to have behavior problems. They often get into trouble in school, have difficulty making friends and getting along with the other children, and come to think of themselves as failures. They are frequently separated into special classes or held back. By the time they reach adolescence, they have little self-esteem, are often on the margins of their peer group, and are at risk of dropping out of school. Unfortunately, those children at greatest risk of having these problems are also the least likely to have access to supports and services that can reduce the risks of damaging long-term outcomes."

According to Daniel, no one ever told him he was learning-disabled: "You're a 'slow learner,' " the teachers had said. Which was different than learning-disabled, as Daniel viewed it. Being a slow learner meant that "it was my fault."

The fact that learning-disabled kids are often blamed for their inability to read, talk, and comprehend normally, represents a great failing in our national educational philosophy, says Dr. Silver. He has asked teachers on numerous occasions, "How many of you would flunk a cerebral palsy kid because he couldn't run the hundred-yard dash in a reasonable period of time?"

The educators will laugh, Silver says, until he asks the next question: "Then why do you penalize learning-disabled children, just because their disability is not visible?" In more than twenty-five years of working with learning-disabled children, says Silver, "I have yet to meet a kid who got up in the morning and said, 'I want to be dumb,' or 'I want to be stupid,' or 'I want to be bad.' The children simply cannot help themselves."

PART TWO

Terri

5

WESTERN PSYCH is a nondescript, seventeen-story building that sits on the Pitt campus in the middle of "Cardiac Hill," so named because of the heightened heart rate of anyone who attempts to climb to the top. Five world-class hospitals and a number of prominent institutes and programs are adjacent to Western Psych, including the largest organ-transplant center in the world. Pitt Stadium, a 50,000-seat fishbowl where the Panthers play football, and Fitzgerald Field House, the basket-ball complex, are also on Cardiac Hill, directly above Western Psych. Other athletic facilities are at the summit, as is a series of new town-houselike dwellings: fraternity row. Here, too, is where Pittsburgh's Hill District begins, the run-down ghetto neighborhood on which Steven Bochco modeled his award-winning television series "Hill Street Blues." Bochco graduated from Pittsburgh's Carnegie-Mellon University, a short walk from Cardiac Hill.

Western Psych possesses a special and shadowed aura for longtime Pittsburghers—a place to avoid at all costs. When I was a boy, my friends and I were warned repeatedly by teachers and parents that if we did not behave, they would send us to Western Psych, an admonition we took seriously. In the 1940s and 1950s, Western Psych was a highly regarded center for the study and practice of psychoanalysis, but by the early 1960s, its reputation was on the wane. In 1972, Thomas E. Detre, chairman of the Department of Psychiatry at Yale University, was appointed chairman of Pitt's Department of Psychiatry and director of Western Psych to inject new life into the facility before it literally faded away. At the time, its operating budget was a little more than $6 million, while less than $200,000 had been generated the prior year for research activities.

Born and raised in Budapest, Detre's enduring and persistent character was formed during the Nazi holocaust; twenty-two members of his family perished in the concentration camps. He alone escaped detection while secretly attending medical school classes. In 1947, unimpressed with Hungary's new Communist leadership, he fled to Rome, where he finished medical school in 1952. Although he is described by friends as down-to-earth and straightforward, his distinctive old-world accent, enhanced by his slow and careful speech, as if he actually analyzes each sentence before uttering it, leads people to suspect that something eerie and sinister lurks behind much of what he does and says. A chain-smoker, Detre will tear away the filter tip of his low-tar cigarette before stuffing its ragged end into an ivory-colored holder, which he waves flamboyantly as he speaks.

In 1960, he introduced a psychiatric inpatient unit at Yale–New Haven Hospital known as Tompkins I, specifically designed for short-term treatment of psychiatric disorders—then a unique concept. This may have been a beginning step toward deinstitutionalization. "In the sixties," Detre explained, "there was a notion that patients had to be hospitalized for long periods of time and receive intensive individual attention in an effort to reconstitute the personality. We adopted a philosophy that the most important thing was to restore social competency in our patients." As a result, Tompkins I was set up as a therapeutic community in which the patients learned to govern themselves. Also pioneered at Tompkins I was the "open unit"—the staff did not lock the doors, the patients did. Some experts considered Tompkins I revolutionary, while others were critical because of its heavy emphasis on a combination of psychiatric medications and demanding, behavior-oriented techniques, criticisms which might easily also apply to Western Psych today.

Within a few years of arriving in Pittsburgh, Detre had recruited to Western Psych most of the up-and-coming "stars" whom he had taught and trained at Yale—dubbed "the Yale Mafia" by resentful old-line Western Psych colleagues. He was constantly on the lookout for young scientists with a strong commitment to original ideas and would provide seed money for their work for the first couple of years until they received independent funding. He then introduced a uniquely corporate practice of granting "bonuses" to scientists who brought research money to the institution. Although his tactics were successful, he has been accused of being Machiavellian; for him, the ends will always justify the means. He has also been likened to an insecure military commander who demands complete obedience and total control.

In 1990, Western Psych's annual operating budget exceeded $110 million. In addition to being supported by a number of prestigious private funding agencies, Western Psych receives more federal funds for psychiatric research than any other institution in the U.S.—more than $13 million annually. Detre was appointed Executive Vice President of Health Sciences at Pitt, a position that makes him responsible for the entire medical complex—40 percent of all the university facilities and student body—a rare and powerful position to be held by a psychiatrist. Today, Western Psych is a nationally renowned Mecca of psychiatric research.

SIXTEEN-YEAR-OLD Terri was the first patient I met at Western Psych, long before I came to know the Scanlon family. Her psychiatrist, medical director of the Adolescent Affective Disorders Unit, 3 West, Boris Birmaher (referred to by staff and patients as "Dr. Boris"), was born and educated in Colombia, and spent his subsequent medical residency in Israel. Usually he is easygoing, but when he becomes angry, his eyes flash and he begins to talk even faster than usual, indicting the system and the limits it imposes, thus impeding his ability to treat "the kids."

When I first met Dr. Boris, he was adamant in his insistence that I understand that most of the kids at Western Psych "are not crazy, but they don't have luck. The kids we admit here are mostly born to lose."

He is referring to the fact that the children on 3 West are primarily economically deprived and have been born into families with histories of mental illness, as well as of neglect and abuse. "It's like a person born with diabetes. They can't be blamed for their illness." He is a short, balding man with a slender frame, cultivating a premature middle-aged paunch. "We can treat our patients, but we can't often cure them."

This is part of the futility of his profession, especially prevalent at an institution such as Western Psych, which is forced to attempt hurried solutions for a large and diverse population. "When a person has cancer, they receive protection and support and basically unlimited treatment. When a person is schizophrenic, they are abandoned by the system— and by all of the people around them."

Even the families of the children who are being treated are hostile. Emotionally disturbed children, especially from low-income populations in which the family unit may not be intact, may first come to the attention of authorities of the juvenile justice system or child welfare agencies, whom they quickly learn to mistrust. For a variety of reasons, including their ongoing resentment toward authority, families may not distinguish between public welfare officials—who may often police them—and doctors who attempt to care for them. Because they live under pressured and tenuous conditions, they are also very private people. "They don't want you to get involved in their personal problems," said Dr. Boris. Meanwhile, no matter what miracles he and his staff may perform, the kids have to return to the same neighborhoods or group homes and in some cases "the same abusive parental situation that made them this way in the first place."

Dr. Boris draws an interesting contrast. The poor people in the Colombian mountains where he traveled by horseback twice a month as part of his medical internship have corn, beans, milk, and eggs to eat, and radios for entertainment. By virtue of the fact that they expect so much less than poor Americans—they don't care about movies, clothes, and cars—they are more content than the poor people in America. Emigrating to America, he expected great enlightenment in psychiatric medicine, but he was sent to a state hospital for children in New York. "Most of the teachers were extremely unqualified. The building was dirty. The smell of urine pervaded the entire institution."

What I found interesting about Western Psych is that many professionals seem to embrace the frustration and futility of their clinical work as if they were a precondition to their efforts. They are perfectly willing to work twelve hours a day, six days a week, with great energy, enthusiasm, and humor. But they know—and they want you to know—that they are attempting to achieve what is nearly impossible. Their impotence makes failure palatable and success, which will infrequently occur, especially exhilarating. Like the smoke jumpers who attack raging forest fires with the knowledge that the fire has its own life, so psychiatrists approach mental illness; the best anyone can often do is prevent the flames from spreading, while waiting for the fire to destroy the forest or burn itself out. This doesn't diminish the firefighters' or the psychiatrists' commitment. It does reduce expectations—and perhaps the pressure that goes along with them. Psychiatrists involved in research with a minimum of clinical involvement and psychiatrists in private practice, whose patients are more genteel and perhaps less critical, are much more optimistic than those who administer to the public sector.

Dr. Boris first began treating Terri at Mayview, a large state-operated psychiatric facility for chronically ill patients in western Pennsylvania, a little less than two years ago. "When I met Terri, she was extremely depressed. She would sit and stare in anger, repeating 'I don't have anything to say.' I spent the first six or seven months gaining her trust. I treated her with many medications and with psychotherapy twice a week. And now she is able to express some of her feelings, although she is more direct and honest in her journal." In order to earn privileges, patients on 3 West and in most other similar institutions must keep a daily diary. "She has more insight when she sits down and writes.

"Terri is one of the most difficult patients I have ever had because she has two major psychiatric disorders. She is bipolar or manic-depressive, and very resistant to treatment, but also she has a severe personality disorder, borderline personality, which by itself is extremely difficult to treat." According to DSM-IIIR, the American Psychiatric Association's (APA) 567-page *Diagnostic and Statistical Manual of Mental Disorders, Third Edition, Revised*, assembled by groups of specialists in different disciplines as an encyclopedia of psychiatric problems, "The essential feature of this disorder is a pervasive pattern of instability of self-image, interpersonal relationships, and mood." It is characterized, among other things, by impulsivity, instability, intense anger, recurrent suicidal threats, chronic feelings of emptiness or boredom. In addition, Terri is a victim of post—traumatic stress disorder (PTSD) in response to an early event, probably sexual abuse, which she is generally unwilling to discuss.

"Terri experiences nightmares, flashbacks, perhaps of rape, and that's the reason she doesn't trust anyone, mainly males. At age two, she was taken away from her parents and has been in multiple foster homes in which we believe she was also abused. On top of this, she is developing bulimia and symptoms of anorexia. Whenever she has the opportunity, she goes to the toilet and vomits. We don't allow her to go to the bathroom by herself, but she looks for places like garbage cans and paper cups to 'purge.' She is also a self-mutilator. Take a look at her arms. They were once bloody all over. When she feels really depressed, she sits in a fetal position for seven or eight hours a day, searching for opportunities to hurt herself. Her mother was psychotic and she married a man who was abusive. Terri's life has been a mess." Dr. Boris shakes his head and whispers, as if he is reluctant to allow anyone else to hear him confess his frustration: "A very difficult case."

Terri is of medium height, with long, unkempt brown hair. When she speaks, she toys with her hair, her clothes, or the bedclothes, refusing to look directly at the person with whom she is conversing. When her symptoms are muted, she will flash a quick and winning smile, with a shy, magnetic quality. When she is frightened or angry, the whites of her eyes become fiery and her body grows rigid, like that of an animal being stalked, ready to strike at anyone venturing near her.

Dr. Boris tells me that Terri has lived in a number of foster homes, and would have preferred to have remained in some of them, but frequent psychiatric-hospital admissions have made stability impossible. Throughout the interview, Terri laughs and giggles nervously.

"I get really depressed, hopelessly depressed," Terri told us that day. "Nothing's ever going to change. I'd be better off dead when I get depressed. I have very bad mood swings."

"What about your appetite?"

"I have no appetite."

"How's your sleep?"

"I don't sleep."

"How's your motivation?"

"I don't have any. It's very hard to do anything like put on makeup or do my hair."

"Do you care what you look like?" asks Dr. Boris.

"I usually don't care about anything," she says. "I have scratched my arms and cut my wrists more than once."

"Did you really mean to kill yourself?"

"I don't know." She shrugs.

"Can you watch movies when you're depressed?"

"I can't watch anything."

"Do you think the ECT is helping you?" Terri has been transferred to Western Psych from Mayview in order to receive electroconvulsive therapy.

"I think it has started to help; the side effects are bad. Headaches and stomachaches that last all day."

"What about memory?"

"There are little things that I don't remember."

"Suppose your depression never comes back. What will you want to do?"

"Go to a group home or a foster home," she says.

"What will you do when you finish school?"

"I want to be a psychiatric nurse or a lawyer."

Dr. Boris tells me that Terri has been in too many foster homes and that she has formed attachments and then had to break those attachments, which has been harmful. Child welfare agencies frequently transfer foster children for just such reasons, although in many cases the "medicine" is more destructive than the "ailment" (attachment) it is designed to prevent. "Terri hopes to become a nurse, and it's no wonder. This is the only positive image she's ever had."

Initially, Terri had responded well to ECT treatment, and in a rare moment the nurses and doctors on 3 West were hopeful. But barely two weeks after being transferred back to Mayview, as an interim to a group home transfer, Terri had fallen apart. Mayview was hardly an ideal setting to provide for a smooth and comfortable transition to a more normal and less restrictive atmosphere, which had been Dr. Boris's goal; in fact, it influenced a reversion to her past behaviors. One of the many failings of the child mental health system is the lack of community-based support, such as a transitional center that would have enhanced Terri's confidence and helped her cope with the challenges of the future. Instead, she was returned to the hotbed of her worst memories. As Dr. Boris had pointed out, even when true progress with a patient is possible, the authorities invariably return his patients to the scene of the crime without having made any attempt to improve the place or situation so that it might be a more suitable, welcoming atmosphere.

When I next saw Terri, three months after she had been returned to Mayview, I had been observing in the Western Psych emergency room, the Diagnostic Evaluation Center, better known as "the DEC," in order to gain an understanding of the many challenges psychiatry faces and the vast array of patients with whom staff must deal on a regular basis. The resident or house doctor on the DEC that evening, Petronilla Vaulx-Smith, was paged at 9:30 P.M., after a relatively quiet night.

Vaulx-Smith is short and slender, with graying hair, thick and dull like steel wool, and narrow fingers whose nails have been gnawed down to tiny pink stubs. Phoning the paging operator, Vaulx-Smith was connected to a charge nurse on 3 West who described a sixteen-year-old girl with a history of self-abuse, who was scratching her arms and banging her head against the wall. The nurse wanted Vaulx-Smith to help initiate a #302, involuntary commitment, and inject her with Thorazine to tranquilize her. The girl would not permit anyone to come close enough to inject her or even talk with her, however. I recognized Terri's description immediately and asked to come along.

Voluntary status is given when the patient or parent/guardian signs forms and agrees to treatment. A voluntary patient can decide to leave, despite a doctor's wishes. Involuntary status is assigned when a patient who needs treatment refuses it. Papers are filed (which is what Petronilla Vaulx-Smith was asked to do for Terri) and a hearing is scheduled within five days to confirm or deny the doctor's actions. Although a voluntary patient may choose to leave the hospital, three days must elapse before he or she can actually depart, during which time doctors may put the patient on involuntary status.

We left the DEC and walked past the security office to a bank of elevators. The main outside door to the facility was to our left, locked at 10 P.M., open only to patients willing to submit to a security check with a metal detector—generally a deterrent to homeless people. A clerk stationed at the desk triggers an emergency calling device which summons the elevator. "Take us to three," Petronilla Vaulx-Smith said, as she fumbled with her key chain. This is a familiar sound at Western Psych—the jingle of keys, followed by the click of a latch, followed by a loud thump, as each door automatically closes and locks behind you. Patient "elopement" is a constant problem.

When we arrived on 3 West perhaps ten seconds later, the charge nurse was waiting, as were two "safety" officers, who fell in step behind us. We were directed to the seclusion room, also called the time-out room or the quiet room, where children are sent when they misbehave. An open time-out (OTO) with the door open is for minor problems, spitting, kicking, etc. A locked time-out (LTO) occurs in response to serious infractions and acts of aggression, with a staff member stationed outside, observing through a window. "Sometimes, kids are not too nice to themselves in the quiet room," says 3 West nurse Wendy Nuss. "There will be head banging or crashing into the walls." Patients will have their shoes and belts removed, as well as barrettes and earrings. Shirts may be confiscated because "kids like to make them into nooses."

No one I have talked to debates the need for such a place in a psychiatric hospital for both kids and adults; tantrums, rages, uncontrolled behavior of any kind, can become quickly infectious. The seclusion area isolates the child, while providing him or her with an opportunity to "think things over." This is the normal approach to behavioral control on 3 West and most other child and adolescent units. Patients are afforded the maximum amount of freedom the staff believes they can handle. If they live up to the staff's expectations, more freedom and more privileges are possible. If they cannot or will not respond, privileges are taken away. Although threats of mass violence or revolt hardly ever occur, there is a "shut down" policy for emergency situations in which the lights are dimmed and patients are confined to their rooms where nurses and doctors can deal with them individually until the crisis has subsided.

Terri was huddled in the far corner of the room, a small, cold, windowless space the size of a walk-in closet, with no furniture and a cement floor. Her long brown hair partially concealed her arms, which were seemingly wrapped around her shoulders. Vaulx-Smith approached Terri hesitantly, while Terri stared woodenly not at her—but through her. "Terri," she said. "What's the matter?"

Terri did not answer. Vaulx-Smith gently placed her hands on Terri's shoulders. But then, as Terri's arms moved, Vaulx-Smith quickly sized up the situation and backed off. "She's got something wrapped around her neck," Vaulx-Smith said. "It's a shoelace." We discovered later that Terri had knotted two thick white laces together.

Vaulx-Smith did not know Terri, and although a child-psychiatric resident, she has spent very little time on any of the child units during her training—a point of contention and debate among many psychiatric educators. Standard practice is to train the resident in general psychiatry first, for at least two years, before permitting regular rotation in a child unit. This may seem logical, but it is also detrimental to the profession. After two years on the front lines of mental illness, confronting geriatrics, schizophrenics, and borderline personalities, young doctors may forget children and lose enthusiasm for psychiatry, preferring to return to the more traditional and "scientific" norms of medicine. Vaulx-Smith has admitted that her enthusiasm is rapidly waning.

The two safety officers walked slowly into the seclusion room and stood in front of Terri. They did not speak. They were waiting, hoping that the girl would give up without a fight. One of the men, tall and wiry, slowly removed his eyeglasses and tucked them into his back pocket, while the other officer, with light brown, slicked-back hair, arms folded across his chest, rocked on his heels. They did not carry weapons.

"Terri, we want to give you something that will relax you," Vaulx-Smith said. "Terri," she said, "c'mon, now." Terri scrunched even farther into the corner. Her arms moved again, and the shoelaces cut a taut white line into her neck. Now the safety officers moved forward. It never occurred to me to consider shoelaces dangerous "contraband," but they were clearly interfering with her breathing. The kids on 3 West are ingenious in the ways they attempt to hurt themselves. A few days ago, a patient swallowed a handful of staples scooped from a unit clerk's desk.

Terri looked beyond the safety officers and Vaulx-Smith, and her eyes latched onto me. For a moment, she related me to Dr. Boris, a physician who could help her escape the nurses who wanted to sedate her and the officers who planned to hold her down. "Please," she whispered. But I was helpless to respond, so she snapped her head back to address the safety officers who had approached her. "Get away from me." The safety officers paused, then moved forward again. "Get away from me," she said, as they surrounded her.

"Terri," said Vaulx-Smith. "Please."

Suddenly, Terri was on her feet, struggling with the safety officers who were attempting to contain her. "You're hurting me! You're hurting me!" Her screams echoed outside in the corridor, where a nurse ordered a curious child, peeking into the doorway, "Go back where you belong."

Considering the onslaught of Terri's attack, the safety officers were gentle, holding her arms and legs and lowering her carefully to the floor. Terri wouldn't give up the shoelaces, however, and the struggle went on for ten or fifteen seconds. Then finally she relented, dropping to the cement with a sickening thud.

Standing behind me, Petronilla Vaulx-Smith emitted a deep breath, almost a gasp, and I turned to look at her. Her face was white, while her eyes shone. "I have never seen a 'take-down' before." She ran a nail-bitten hand through her long, graying hair. Color flooded to her cheeks, revealing a momentary smile of relief. "I guess these things aren't supposed to bother me, but seeing it for the first time scares me to death."

Later, I learn that although Vaulx-Smith had not witnessed a "take-down," she had recently cared for a boy whose leg had been fractured after a "take-down" in this same unit. Vaulx-Smith admits to a certain hostility toward the safety officers because of this experience—until now. "I guess they did their best with Terri, and I can understand how injuries happen, despite how gentle you try to be. But why not put carpet on the seclusion room floor? I know it is more difficult to maintain than cement, considering the potential vomit and blood, but for God's sake, these kids are incredibly fragile."

A nurse appeared with a hypodermic needle. The safety officers momentarily contained Terri's thrashing legs. As the Thorazine was injected, Terri abruptly stopped fighting; she knew she was beaten. "Now get away from me," she said. "Haven't all of you hurt me enough?" Terri was upset, but was not crying; she had learned long ago the futility of her tears.

6

IN RETROSPECTIVE STUDIES of more than 2,000 death certificates of people who committed suicide in western Pennsylvania, David Brent, Chief, Division of Child and Adolescent Psychiatry at Western Psych, discovered that the suicide rate has been "low and constant" for 10- to 14-year-olds, but over the past three decades, the suicide scenario has "tripled" for kids 15 through 19, while the rate for the general population has remained steady. The potential for a rapid increase in suicide among young people is very high, says Brent: Only 10 of every 100,000 children and adolescents are actually successful at committing suicide, "but there are 1,000 *attempted* suicides annually of each 100,000 children and young adults, ages thirteen to twenty-four."

Most suicide attempters are females or nonwhite males, while most suicide completers are white males. The number of attempters increases with age, peaking around thirty-five, while completers increase over their life span—from young to old. Says Brent, "The majority of attempts are impulsive and only about a third who attempt actually want to die." More planning is evident for kids who complete suicide, "such as tying weights to your legs when attempting to drown yourself." Complet-

ers' notes indicate that they are "sorry, but can't stand living anymore."
In order of success, the agents of doom are firearms, hanging, carbon
monoxide, and drug overdose. For those who don't succeed, the most
popular methods are drugs and self-mutilation. One tenth of the attempters will try again, 10 percent of whom will eventually be successful. "There is a crescendo effect." Kids begin modestly, learn what does
not work, then try again with more lethal methods. More white males
are successful because of their familiarity with firearms and the availability of firearms in their home.

"We also found a synergistic relationship between alcohol intoxica-
tion and the use of firearms." Slightly intoxicated kids were about twice
as likely to kill themselves with a gun, while those highly intoxicated
were seven times more likely. Contrary to public opinion, suicide, the
second leading cause of death among 15- to 29-year-olds, is traced not to
the breakdown of the family structure, but more to feelings of hopelessness for the future.

A most interesting aspect of Brent's work concerns the relationship
between suicide and psychiatric disorder. A primary concept of many
suicide-prevention programs is that "suicide is not associated with
mental illness, but it is really erroneous information." Ninety percent
of Brent's completed suicide victims had at least one diagnosable
psychiatric disorder. "In fact, most of the kids we studied had been
chronically psychiatrically ill for at least seven years at the time of
their demise."

Another telling finding is that teenage suicide can be contagious.
More significant for teenagers than "genetic loading" is "exposure" to
people who had committed suicide, especially a family member or close
friend. Brent says that schools, in their zeal to help and to support
grieving students, often take action which enhances rather than dimin-
ishes the possibility of an outbreak of teenage suicide. He advises
against memorial services for kids who commit suicide or discussion
groups about the child "because you end up exposing the suicidal
behavior to people who are very peripheral, and we know that there is a
'modeling effect.' "

Psychiatrists who have studied suicide in children and adults stress
repeatedly that the best way to begin preventing suicide when "ideation"

is suspected is to bring the subject up. According to Brent, "It's important to clarify and discuss all talk of suicide or wanting to die. Whenever suicide is a possibility, you should be asking these kids, 'Are you thinking about hurting yourself or wanting to die?' "

Initially, Brent's assessment didn't make sense to me. If nurses and psychiatrists at Western Psych did not want to expose suicidal behavior to kids and adults who are very peripheral because of a "modeling" effect, then wasn't it possible that persistent questioning and probing about suicide were more likely to enhance than prevent the suicide from occurring in vulnerable and suggestive people? My question was answered one day on the DEC, after observing a young man whom I will call Augie.

Early one winter morning, Augie walked into the DEC and surrendered to a safety officer the contents of his pockets, among them a long, bone-handled hunting knife in a leather sheath. The knife was placed in a manila envelope for safekeeping while all other possessions—wallet, change, keys—were immediately returned to him. Then the charge nurse, Mary Grace Fitzgerald, a pleasant, efficient veteran, ushered Augie into a tiny "triage" room for a preliminary interview. A "body beeper," which can emit a silent distress signal to the safety officer, was tucked into her pocket. "What brings you to the DEC, Augie?"

In a halting but clearly presented narrative, Augie, who was wearing a black Ninja-type suit with blue designs, black loafers, and a Timex wristwatch, briefly described his family problems: the death of his brother, now nearly a year ago; mounting bills; arguments with his girlfriend. Nodding and noting this information on the printed form in her clipboard, Mary Grace Fitzgerald asked: "Have you ever thought about killing yourself?"

"I've thought about not wanting to wake up."

"Have you thought about killing somebody else?"

"Yes, but no one in particular."

Mary Grace Fitzgerald escorted Augie into the waiting area. Shuffling slowly, not unlike an inmate in a chain gang, he sank resignedly into a chair, staring idly at his image as reflected off the one-way glass. In the office behind that glass, Fitzgerald compared the process of interviewing her patients to reading "a really good short story. I listen to the best literature in the world two or three times a day." At that moment, a buzzer sounded from the ambulance or "back porch" entrance of the DEC. Most likely, the police were bringing in a patient. Fitzgerald picked up her body beeper and excused herself. "They're playing my song," she said.

Because Western Psych is a teaching facility, part of the University of Pittsburgh School of Medicine, it is standard operating procedure to provide psychiatric residents with maximum hours of patient contact. Thus, although Fitzgerald might have conducted the evaluation which normally follows all triaging procedures, Augie was made to wait for the arrival of Nate Daubner (a pseudonym), a second-year resident on DEC rotation. While gulping a quick cup of coffee, Daubner examined Mary Grace Fitzgerald's report and asked a few preliminary questions concerning Augie's general state of mind. Opening the manila envelope and lifting gingerly with thumb and forefinger Augie's surrendered hunting knife, Daubner, a balding, well-dressed doctor, observed: "Never can tell when you might need to skin a rabbit."

A few minutes later in an examination room, Augie explained to Daubner that his brother had died a little less than a year ago. "I think about it every day." He pressed his fingers up against his forehead and temples, as if to hold back a threatening wellspring of tears. "I wish it had been me." Daubner probed in a number of different directions, attempting to determine the depth of Augie's relationship with his brother, the extent of Augie's feelings of guilt regarding the death, the frequency of his interactions with parents and siblings.

Daubner, who has a soft, mellow voice and who nods encouragingly and listens carefully, wanted to know why Augie had picked this particular morning to make an appearance at the DEC, especially considering all the months that had elapsed since his brother's death. "My mood changes," said Augie. One minute he would be quiet and contented, and the next minute he'd become angry and unpredictable. Occasionally, he had trashed the apartment where he and his girlfriend lived, destroyed furniture—for no particular reason. "It just happens," Augie said.

Augie had been a frequent visitor to the emergency room of his local hospital, complaining of chest pains and related physical ailments; he had had repeated dreams of menacing people sneaking into his apartment and attacking him. His father had died about ten years ago, and one of his mother's two brothers had been institutionalized for emotional problems. Augie did not know what he expected the doctors to do for him at Western Psych. In response to Daubner's next question, Augie admitted: "Yes, I think about death a lot."

Even though Augie was openly cooperative, I initially had my doubts about what seemed to be the clinician's central focus: an ongoing search for "suicide ideation." Almost anyone, in moments of anxiety, might have idly pondered the notion of taking a life—his own or someone else's. That very day a friend had observed that she frequently contemplated bashing her mother's head in with a sledgehammer. She was laughing about it, but she too might have confessed that thought under similarly stressed circumstances in the emergency room of a psychiatric institution.

"I understand that you know better and that you feel completely in control," Daubner said to Augie. "But imagine, just for a minute, if you were really serious about suicide, how would you do it?"

Augie looked down at his feet. "Poison or something. Maybe Clorox to drink." Daubner made note of Augie's answer on a yellow legal pad. The specificity of the response will not strike home until later.

Throughout the interview I waited for Daubner to ask Augie why he carried a hunting knife in the middle of the city. Later, Daubner admitted that it would have been a perfectly reasonable question had it occurred to him. But he confessed to a certain "performance anxiety"— being observed by an outsider while interviewing a patient, an unusual situation—which had made him exceedingly nervous.

I find it comforting and reassuring to know that psychiatrists suffer from the same feelings of insecurity as we common folks—perhaps more. This is probably because they have been attempting to understand—or question—the human condition more than most other people and have recognized the futility of such an enterprise. I have written about surgeons for many years and very rarely have I heard any surgeon admit to feelings of doubt or low self-esteem. Not that a surgeon cannot cry and feel remorse after losing a patient or botching a procedure, or experience loneliness and isolation. But they learn early the necessity of developing an implacable facade and maintaining a distanced clinical perspective. A transplant surgeon once told me that he had accepted the fact that he could save the lives of only 80 percent of his patients. "If you happen to be one of those 20 percent who do not make it, it's just not my fault."

Psychiatrists and psychiatric nurses, on the other hand, often seem to think that whatever bad things happen to their patients are always their fault, even when they aren't, even when there is absolutely nothing that could have been done to prevent a situation from taking place. RN Annette Baughman was sweating out such a situation at the very moment we were discussing Augie.

The day before, a man in his late twenties had wandered into the DEC, distraught. A well-known professional athlete who lived in Pittsburgh, he explained to Baughman that his wife had left him, his finances were in a state of ruin, and he was unemployed. He assumed blame for all of the bad things that had happened to him. For the past two months, he had locked himself in his house, drinking beer and refusing to answer the telephone. His only contact was with his family, who checked on him periodically by rapping persistently on his door until he answered. Now he was ready to try to get back on his feet. Coming to the DEC had been the first and hardest step.

Annette Baughman was moved by this story. "He is a very nice and sincere man," she told me. "And he's desperate to turn his life around." Normally, considering the fact that the man had private insurance, hospital admission would not be a problem, but at the moment the census at Western Psych was 100 percent. So Annette Baughman set about the task of finding a bed for her patient.

After a few phone calls, Baughman located a "research bed" on the eleventh floor, expressly set aside for people with a "first episode" of depression. The fact that the man had been drinking steadily four or five bottles of beer a night was briefly discussed as a possible disqualifying factor, but Baughman assured the medical director, whom she had contacted at home, that the patient had used alcohol only very recently and only to help himself sleep. "This is clean depression," she assured him, no substance abuse involved. The medical director subsequently agreed, and she contacted the charge nurse on the unit to ready the bed for admission.

Perhaps only thirty minutes had passed, but by the time Annette Baughman returned to the waiting area with the paperwork complete, ready for signature, the man was standing at the reception area, explaining that he had changed his mind. "I need to go home and take care of a few things. I'll be back in two days." He looked at the date on his wristwatch. "Monday."

"We don't know if there'll be a bed for you on Monday," Baughman said.

"Then call me. I'll take the first bed available after Monday."

"But will you be safe? That's the most important thing. We don't want you to hurt yourself."

"I hope so."

"Well, you are going to have to give me more assurance than that."

"That's all I can tell you. What else can I say?"

"There's a bed available for you right now," Baughman said. "But you'll lose it if you walk out."

"Believe me," the man said. "I want to come in here a lot more than you want me to come in, but I can't."

"You want us to contact your family and tell them that we are concerned?"

Suddenly the man began to cry. "It was so hard to come here," he said, pausing. "Some folks simply don't understand. You know that? It's like talkin' to yourself."

"If you can't handle the pain, don't go," said Baughman. "Stay. We can talk all night."

The man shook his head and dabbed his eyes with his sleeve. "I'll be back."

The following afternoon, the man's sister telephoned the hospital looking for her brother. When the switchboard operator could not locate him, the call was transferred to the DEC, which is the port of entry for most Western Psych patients. Annette Baughman took the call. The man had contacted his sister yesterday evening to tell her he was being admitted, she learned. Thus the family had not been worried—in fact, they had been relieved when he did not return home.

But now, he had been missing for twenty-four hours. "I should have never let him go," Baughman said. Periodically, for the rest of the evening, she would repeat, "I keep thinking about that man. What have I done?"

BEFORE ENDING HIS interview with Augie, Nate Daubner requests permission to contact Augie's girlfriend, Maddie, who is at work, and Augie recites the telephone number while Daubner writes it down. Nate Daubner knows that some of the symptoms to which Augie has alluded—chest pains, rapid heartbeat, paranoid visions—are those most associated with cocaine, but the fact that Augie has agreed to allow Daubner to call a friend or family member indicates that substance abuse is probably not Augie's problem.

Sitting at a tiny desk tucked behind the one-way glass, Daubner places a call to Maddie, who, he is told by her supervisor, is on her break. Fifteen minutes later, he calls again, but she has still not returned. He declines to identify himself, but promises to try again soon. In the interim, Nate Daubner leans back in his chair and ponders his patient's story. Augie is articulate and calm, especially compared to the general hysteria witnessed on the DEC on a regular basis; he is a guy attempting to maintain control. What are the chances he can continue to exert control—and straighten out his problems without institutionalized intervention, meaning hospital admission? Daubner furrows his brow. It would not be an outlandish suggestion, if such were a possibility, to call for a consultation from Inspector Poirot. Psychiatry may be a science, but it is rooted in the nuts and bolts of detection.

Meanwhile, Annette Baughman has embarked upon her own whodunit (or "whodunwhat"?) of the day. A sixty-five-year-old woman is deposited at the DEC by two police officers, summoned by her daughter, who maintained that her mother was attempting to kill herself by slashing her shins with a razor blade, an accusation that the mother totally disputes. The daughter, who says that her mother has frequently attempted suicide, wants to commit her mother on an involuntary admission. The mother says that this is her daughter's way of removing her from the apartment for which she, *the mother*, pays. Her daughter has launched a vendetta against her because she dislikes the daughter's new boyfriend, a reputed drug dealer. The mother says she wants to kick daughter and boyfriend out of the house.

Daubner explains the tenuous nature of the entire concept of involuntary commitment in Pennsylvania and throughout the U.S. "The law says a person must have endangered his or someone else's life in order to justify commitment to a coroner, ordinarily the final arbiter. A person must have actually *done an act*." How a psychiatrist will phrase the presentation of this "act" will be the determinant factor. Although the law is the same across the state, each coroner's interpretation may be different. In Pittsburgh, the coroner's office is flexible, and will almost always follow the psychiatric recommendation, but in Philadelphia the letter of the law is much more strictly defined, an approach that may protect individual liberties but not without some societal danger.

In an effort to gain insight into the situation, Annette Baughman telephones the woman's son, who lives outside of the home and who disavows any knowledge of his mother's previous suicide attempts or of any psychiatric history, although he knows that his mother has a tendency to drink too much, which often leads to erratic behavior. Baughman telephones the daughter, who reports that her mother removed a razor blade kept in an empty tuna fish can and used normally to cut off her calluses, and held it threateningly against her wrist. The daughter makes it clear that she has no interest in continuing a conversation with Annette Baughman; she wants to talk with her mother. The mother makes it clear she will only talk to Annette Baughman or her son, but never her daughter. Eventually she changes her mind. Baughman transfers the call to the waiting area, where the mother lifts the receiver, listens for fifteen seconds, and then hangs up the phone. Watching through the one-way glass, Baughman says, "This is a bullshit domestic case."

But is it? A resident, newly arrived at the DEC, examines the mother and discovers a number of scars on her wrist and fresh cuts and scratches on her ankles, which, the mother claims, happened when she tripped and fell on a broken drinking glass. He allows the possibility, thus sending Baughman back to the phone to inquire about prior history of suicide attempts. Now the line at the daughter's apartment is busy. A few minutes later, when Baughman tries back, no one answers. She contacts the police dispatcher, who reports that the emergency medical technicians who had first arrived on the scene testified that the mother had seemed intent upon hurting herself. Annette Baughman is also informed that the police had originally transported the woman to the emergency room at a nearby medical facility, where she was interviewed by a social worker who determined that she would be better served at Western Psych.

Baughman phones the emergency room and is told that the social worker is en route home for the night. She obtains the social worker's home number, waits fifteen minutes, then phones, catching the social worker as she comes in. Listening to the social worker's version of the incident, Baughman becomes convinced that the daughter's story is more accurate, until the social worker informs her, near the end of the conversation, that all of her information comes from the daughter. "It's going to take ten hours to figure this whole thing out," Annette Baughman says.

Baughman telephones the daughter, who now answers the phone and who angrily paraphrases her story, admitting that she and her mother had been drinking beer since eleven o'clock that morning. Baughman telephones the woman's son, who offers to come and get his mother and kick his sister out of his mother's apartment. "This goes on and on," Baughman says.

"I see no reason for this woman to be admitted," Annette Baughman tells the resident. "This is Saturday. The daughter cannot petition the court for an involuntary until Monday, which means, even if the judge disallows, she'll be here for two nights."

"I don't think we need to keep her here as long as she has another place to go," the resident agrees. "Her son will come and get her."

"You try to be a patient advocate," says Annette Baughman, "but in the end, it's so much easier to admit them to the hospital and let the courts work it out."

Although Baughman's statement sounds spontaneously flip, she has struck an unfortunately accurate chord, one that is especially troublesome in the child and adolescent mental health system. Private non-profit hospitals such as Western Psych, along with hundreds of for-profit institutions across the U.S., have become the de facto emergency treatment centers for most Americans, especially the urban poor like Augie, Terri, and Daniel, because there are no other alternatives.

It is quite possible that Baughman's patient and her daughter could have solved their problems had a social worker been available to mediate their dispute. If the woman is admitted to Western Psych for the five days it takes to submit and obtain a ruling from a family court judge, charges of perhaps as much as $5,000 will be assessed. State Medicare will assume responsibility for some of that coverage, while Western Psych will be forced to shoulder the remaining costs.

7

AS ANNETTE BAUGHMAN continues to find her way through the complicated mother-daughter-son/alcoholic web, Nate Daubner has presented what he does and doesn't know about Augie's case to the attending physician on duty, Gregory Supolsky.

This illustrates one of the inexplicable riddles of health-care management in psychiatry specifically and in medicine generally. During the day, a full complement of experienced physicians and social workers are in charge of each and every unit, including the DEC. A patient who wanders in from 8:00 A.M. to 6:00 P.M. or thereabouts may be attended by a nurse or resident supervised by a more senior staffer, such as Supolsky. The same patient stumbling in at 9:00 P.M. will not receive such supervised attention—at least not initially. Nate Daubner, Petronilla Vaulx-Smith, or any of twenty-five residents will serve alone as "house doctor" beginning early in the evening and on through the night.

"What is it?" asks Supolsky. In his role as a teacher, Supolsky is asking Daubner to name the official diagnosis as listed in DSM-IIIR, a prerequisite for reimbursement from third-party payers such as Medicare, the "Blues," or other health-care insurance.

"Major death, single episode, nonpsychotic," Daubner replies.

"So what do you want to do?" Supolsky means: Shall Augie be admitted or assigned outpatient treatment?

"I don't know," says Daubner. "I could go either way."

They agree that Augie is in the correct "catchment area" for admission. The federal government mandates that psychiatric institutions must admit patients on medical assistance based upon residency. There are three inpatient catchment areas within the Allegheny County limits and dozens of outpatient treatment centers. A hospital floor chart is anchored to the wall above Daubner's desk, listing each unit, the number of beds per unit, and the last name and first initial of each patient. The question of admission is tenuous. From a clinical point of view, Augie is not seriously impaired, but can he or will he wait for Daubner to arrange a referral at an outpatient clinic—a process that may take up to two weeks—or does he want or need help today? Supolsky suggests that they put the question to Augie, and Daubner agrees.

In the examination room, Supolsky asks Augie to tell him in his own words how he feels and the reason he has come to the DEC for treatment. More than two hours have passed since Augie first surrendered his bone-handled knife, and after two previous interviews, it is clear that he has lost his taste for his story. Perhaps he doesn't even believe it anymore. He goes through the motions woodenly, with Supolsky nodding cursorily. When presented with the option of staying or going, he immediately chooses outpatient treatment. Augie's affect has remained glassy-eyed and ambivalent, but upon learning that Daubner never contacted his girlfriend, he begins to sputter and mumble. Nate Daubner doesn't seem to notice Augie's agitation.

The frequency of the phone calls into the DEC seems to diminish as day leads to dusk and darkness, but the intensity of the calls is heightened at night, as illustrated by the various nurses' notations in the DEC telephone log. Most of the inquiries concern children and adolescents.

Unidentified mother calling about 7-year-old child who lies, cheats, sneaks around, breaks fences, suicidal, homicidal. Mother at wits' end.

Unid. mother of 10-year-old, killing animals, one cat, plus several dogs.

21-year-old. Can't stop thoughts of wanting to hurt myself. One of these days, I am going to hang myself.

Man with obsessive thoughts that his friends hate him. Can't stop thinking how much they hate him.

Unid. caller wants to talk. (We talked.)

Unid. caller is gay. Wants to talk. (We talked.)

Unid. woman from West Virginia seeking information for her son, who is a devil worshiper.

Unid. man claims a Krishna gave him cyanide.

Bell Telephone reporting a woman on the line, threatening to kill herself by jumping off the Bell building. [The company traced the call.] She was calling from a pay phone on [Western Psych Unit] 10.

Woman called about her son having nausea, vomiting. Suggested medical consultation.

Woman called again, about husband. Same problem.

Woman called again—for self.

Some of the people who telephone the DEC are regulars. Barney calls with a "thought for the day," while Stanley will telephone about sixty times a week, sometimes with a fake name and disguised voice. Lonely and desperate people, Annette Baughman says. "Some of them you get to know real well, and the regulars will ask you out on dates. This is their second home. I don't mind talking to them, helping to calm them, make them a little happy."

Baughman is going on vacation the following morning. "A cruise in the Bahamas during hurricane season—I'll try anything for a change of pace." She thumbs through the chart of the professional athlete who is missing, while snacking from a box of popcorn and a bag of plump ripe grapes. "Anxiety," she says, eating manically. She cannot stop thinking about what happened to that man. She telephones the man's sister, who has received no word. "This case is going to haunt me. Where could he be? What could he be doing? My imagination is going wild."

I once knew a man who was writing a novel about a reporter working the night shift for United Press International (UPI) who had been tracking the progress of a search for a group of cavers lost in a cavern in the mountains. In contact by telephone, he would receive periodic reports from "stringers" who would interview bystanders and officials on the scene. The reporter would write down the information provided on the telephone, ask a few cursory questions, and immediately type all salient facts into the teletype, which would clatter off in hundreds of cross-country directions. As illuminating as some of the information was, having to do with the geology of the area and the general challenge of caving, the bottom-line message always remained the same: The cavers were missing, and no one knew where they were or how long they had been gone.

For the reporter, sitting alone in the tiny room, the cavers became overpoweringly real. He did not focus his attention upon their rescue, but rather obsessed about their personalities and the state of their being: What were they doing at that particular moment, or saying, or feeling? Were their faces filthy with cave dust? Was the water that they had to drink—if they had water to drink—tepid? Running low? Were they frightened? Did they have confidence in being found? The reporter's sense of reality became increasingly distorted as he plugged away at his teletype in the isolated darkness.

A long silence ensues at the DEC during which everyone focuses upon their ongoing battle against paperwork—until a sudden commotion erupts in the waiting area. "I don't belong here, man. I ain't comin' here. Where's my mom at? Why ain't she comin' here, man? I gotta go to the bathroom!" This comes from a twelve-year-old boy who has been admitted to Western Psych twice before with a diagnosis of "conduct disorder" defined by DSM-IIIR as "a predominance of aggressive physical behavior, usually toward both adults and peers." Tall and slender, with long blond hair and high cheekbones, he is being committed by his mother, who summoned the police to bring him in. (Parents can bypass normal legal procedures for commitment of children fourteen and under.) "I'll kill her for sending me here, I swear to God, I'll kill that bitch."

Quickly sizing up the situation, Annette Baughman directs the safety officers to remove the chairs from the examination room. Distraught patients will often try to escape by throwing a chair through the window. Even now, the boy is pounding his fist up against the glass.

"I want to talk to my mother."

"Not with the statements you just made," says Annette Baughman.

"I'm not going to kill her, I was just talking."

"Well, I don't think she—or we—can trust you."

If there is one basic lesson to learn from working or observing at the DEC, it is pessimism, disbelief, lack of trust in first impressions, or in any impression, in any word or action. Nothing is necessarily what it seems, and no one is necessarily who or what they say they are. Life is up for grabs; the future is as impossible to predict as the past is to define. Annette Baughman has learned that lesson repeatedly, as will Nate Daubner as his residency goes forward.

One of the promises I made to officials at Western Psych when I first approached them for access to the inner workings of the institution was that I would not interfere with physician-patient interaction, even if I believed I could help or disagreed with the actions taken by the clinical staff. For the most part, I honored my pledge. I admired most of the people at Western Psych and respected the science and medicine I was privileged to observe. But sometimes physicians and nurses are either too harried to understand their patients or become too unattached to listen carefully to their patients or decipher the indirect language often communicated. Not that writers (or sociologists or anthropologists) are especially intuitive—but sometimes an objective and distanced observer can make a difference.

After unsuccessfully attempting to contact Augie's girlfriend for more than an hour, Daubner returns momentarily to the waiting area to tell Augie that he is going to proceed with Augie's outpatient referral, just to move the process forward.

"Okay," Augie says. "I understand. But my girlfriend knows me pretty good," he adds.

"I'm sure she does," Daubner says politely.

I had moved to the waiting area in order to watch Augie more closely and to see if he struck up conversations with other people, but when Daubner returns to his desk behind the one-way glass, Augie slumps back down in his chair and begins mumbling. "My girlfriend knows me better than anybody, but if the doctor don't want to call her. . . ." He shrugs. "He's the doctor."

Eventually I say, "The doctor will call your girlfriend; you must push him a little. Tell him it's important."

"My girlfriend knows me better than anyone."

"Tell that to the doctor again; tell him how much you want him to talk to your girlfriend. He's a nice guy; he'll do it."

When Daubner next passes through the waiting area, Augie gets up and taps him on the shoulder. "My girlfriend knows things about me that nobody else does," he says.

"Do you want me to keep trying her?" Daubner asks.

"You're the doctor," says Augie, "whatever you think is best."

Luckily, Daubner decides to try to contact Augie's girlfriend once again. After a brief conversation, he returns to the waiting area and leads Augie back into the examination room. Within a few minutes, Augie is weeping hysterically; within a half hour, Augie is made an inpatient at Western Psych. Nate Daubner learns that Augie had been much more desperate than he or Supolsky had imagined. The thoughts of death—"suicide ideation"—had been quite real. Augie's girlfriend told Daubner that Augie had attempted to drink a glass of Clorox yesterday evening, but she had taken it away from him. He had purchased the hunting knife about a month ago, but lacking the courage to use it on himself, had tried repeatedly to persuade her to stab him in his sleep.

WHILE WRITING ABOUT a children's hospital, I once accompanied a security officer on his graveyard shift—a very lonely experience. There were many children alone in bed, watching TV, cuddling and whispering to stuffed animals in the darkness. Some parents wandered aimlessly through the halls, exhausted but afraid to sleep, while others curled up on chairs and on the floor in corners sneaking cigarettes in unauthorized areas, many softly crying. We went up and down from the eleventh-floor tower to the sub-basement, checking doors, seeking fire hazards, listening to the intermittent crackle of conversation coming from walkie-talkies slipped into our side pockets, as the command center communicated to the other officers on duty.

I remember the intensity of my isolation and sadness at the sight of so many children and frightened parents fighting to maintain composure and steal a few needed hours of sleep through the scary night—until we happened upon a group of residents and nurses huddled around a tray of food rescued from a late-afternoon hospital board meeting. The cheese was old and dry and the crackers were soggy, but for a couple of minutes, we all stood together in the dimly lit hallway, talking and nibbling. I cannot recall a word that was said during that conversation, or who else was there besides myself and the officer on duty, but even now, two years later, the soothing feelings of comfort I derived—a reassuring moment that confirmed our mutual connection to the human race—remain a sharply focused memory.

Such a reaffirmation was rare at Western Psych, because the prognosis for most of the patients is so poor. There are few glimmers of hope to be found through most of the institution, especially for the kids, who are often happiest and safest behind the confines of these locked doors. With the exception of the occasional patient wandering into the DEC or forcibly dragged in by police, nobody stirs in a psychiatric hospital from midnight to 6:00 A.M. Many of the patients have been medicated or are confined to the silence of their spaces. Televisions flicker silently in lounge areas, where night nurses sit stoically, sipping stale coffee and finishing their charting. Now and then you will hear the slam/thunk of a locked door as a nurse or safety officer moves between units, while the main elevator sporadically dashes up and down upon command. But basically there is silence in the night at Western Psych, and within the silence an undeniable gash of loneliness and alienation.

AT ABOUT 6:00 A.M. on the morning after Terri had attempted to hurt herself, I waited until Petronilla Vaulx-Smith decided to creep into a nearby office and attempt to steal an hour of sleep before I made my way back to 3 West before heading home.

Terri was fast asleep. The crisis was over. The nurses were sitting quietly contemplating the dawn and the gray finale of their endless night. One of the nurses showed me a poem that Terri had written that evening.

> I was lost, down
> confused and used

I hated life.
I wanted to die, to have no life.

Later, Dr. Boris told me that if ECT, the new medications he was prescribing, and her ongoing psychotherapy did not begin to make significant impact, then the message inherent in Terri's poem could quite likely come true.

DANIEL

DANIEL WAS FASCINATED by mechanical devices, toasters, televisions, computers, anything electronic. Despite constant warnings, he seemed compelled to take things apart, willy-nilly, and then attempt to put them back together again. Sometimes he didn't know what he was taking apart—or why—and since he didn't know what these devices did or how they worked, returning them to their original state was often far beyond his abilities. Instructional and how-to books were not the answer because he could not read them. There were no friends who shared his interests.

In his room at the group home, Daniel had an array of discarded and outmoded equipment, an old manual typewriter with no ribbon and broken keys, a speedometer from a Volkswagen Rabbit, and various parts from TVs, radios, computers, and VCRs discovered in trash bins. Daniel's goal was to fix all these items so that they worked—or to use all the parts to build his robot. He also had a substantial key collection—perhaps as many as two hundred at any given time—but no idea what locks they might open. Most of his allowance was used to buy locks, chains, and inexpensive battery-operated alarms to protect his key and junk collections. At the group home, Daniel was often robbed of money and clothes, but his keys and "spare parts" were usually safe.

What was most amazing, despite his lack of knowledge, was how many things Daniel could actually and instinctively fix. Whenever the VCR, the TV, the doorbell, the computer, went on the blink, Daniel was often summoned to help—sometimes successfully. He repaired radios, clocks, speakers, lamps. One would think that Daniel's caseworkers would tap into his passion for the way things worked, but never once had he been enrolled in a vocational program or connected with someone who might help maximize his mechanical potential. The home was affiliated with a county summer program which, according to Daniel's caseworker, "kept the boys out of trouble and taught them how to wash cars."

Instead of such a wasteful investment of time, I wanted Daniel to go to summer school and improve his reading skills. I contacted the school district which had authority over Daniel's education. Yes, there was summer school, but because he was a teenager, he would not be permitted to attend second-grade-level reading classes with eight-year-olds. Obviously, it would be useless to take age-appropriate reading classes, for he could not follow the reading or the discussion it triggered. There was little coordination between Daniel's caseworker at his group home, the Children and Youth Services (CYS) caseworker responsible for his disposition, the social worker at his special needs school, and the supervisor at the school board which had sent him to the school. They communicated once a year, a routine thirty-minute interaction.

At the Western Psych library, I found a list of self-help organizations published by the National Institute of Mental Health, which led me to the national headquarters of the Association for Children and Adults with Learning Disabilities, coincidentally located in suburban Pittsburgh. Two telephone calls later, I learned about the Tillotson School for learning-disabled kids, which had a summer program. A letter introducing Daniel to Catherine Tillotson, its founder, led to a personal meeting among the three of us one Saturday morning and a summer scholarship for Daniel. To her credit, Daniel's group home counselor was able to arrange for transportation.

Daniel was excited about attending the Tillotson School, not only because he would receive an hour of individualized instruction in math and reading five days a week, in addition to attending age-appropriate classes, but the kids, as he put it, "were real, like me—not crazy." In a nutshell, this issue of attending school with "normal kids" was the essence of Daniel's problem with the educational system. After being discharged from Mayview State Hospital and transferred to a group home, Daniel had been admitted to Craig House Technoma, which contracted with his school board to educate kids who were retarded, evidenced behavioral problems, or possessed severe learning disabilities—or who manifested a combination of these problems.

Daniel was more than willing to admit to having learning disabilities, but he was adamant in his belief that he did not belong at Craig House because it was for kids "out of control." And because he did not belong, he was not particularly interested in cooperating with his teachers or interacting with fellow students. Thus, his behavior at school was unpredictable; he often became adamant, refusing to do his work, insisting that he was unfairly being treated as a "crazy" kid.

The situation was not cut-and-dry. No, Daniel was not "crazy." Usually, he did not act out and misbehave as did many of the Craig House kids, but he was not always in control, either. The scars of his past would suddenly and mysteriously visit him, causing sadness, depression, and unpredictable resentment toward adults. And because he felt that he was forced to be in an atmosphere in which he did not belong, he responded negatively and sometimes violently to the misbehavior of others.

He experienced delusions of grandeur, in which as a policeman—a super-cop like his mythical hero, Michael Knight—he exerted control over destructive forces in society, and would attempt to interject order in situations that did not involve him. Unlike Michael Knight, Daniel was not only physically smaller than most kids his age, but also timid and afraid of being hurt. When the "crazy" kids took unkindly toward his interference and attacked him, Daniel retreated and often cried. Later, embarrassed by his behavior, he would make up stories of being outnumbered and picked on, but fighting valiantly. A perfect example of Daniel's unpredictable behavioral problems and how the forces in his life exacerbated them occurred one morning in the early spring.

The night before, someone had broken into the office at the group home and stolen approximately fifty dollars in petty cash, used primarily for Saturday-night pizza, skating parties, and transportation for the kids. In the unsupervised atmosphere in which the mob often ruled, Daniel and other residents conducted a room-by-room search for the money, to no avail. Exhilarated by the adrenaline of the mob action, Daniel fell asleep at 4:00 A.M. and was awakened at the usual time, 6:30. Tired and angry, he dressed in summer shorts and a tank top jersey—inappropriate for school, especially in the chilly Pittsburgh spring. It had been thirty-two degrees outside the night before. A staff member told him to change clothes, an order which Daniel bitterly resented. "This is a free country; I'm allowed to wear anything I want."

"Not if you are going to get sick—protecting you from sickness is my responsibility, and you are going to do what I tell you and dress in warmer clothing."

Daniel complied, but the stress of the long night and his resentment at the staff member's interference ate at him on the way to Craig House. During the second period, Joe, a tall, fat boy with severe behavior problems, approached Daniel for money. Joe allegedly had been extorting two dollars a day from Daniel for "protection." This time, Daniel, sullen and angry over what had happened at the home and sick and tired of Joe terrorizing him, suddenly exploded. He began throwing chairs at Joe and yelling and screaming hysterically until teachers pinned him to the ground. Soon after, he was sent to the group home, where he was to remain in his room under observation until he could calm down.

Probably the day would have passed and Daniel would have been able to collect himself if he had been able to tell someone about Joe's relentless extortion (if the extortion had actually taken place). But Daniel went to his room—and was promptly forgotten. A few minutes later, staring straight ahead and angrily muttering to himself, he walked past the front desk and out the front door. Witnesses said that he was screaming as he headed toward the main road, gesturing and cursing and glaring at the ground, but no one tried to stop him.

Looking neither to his left nor his right, he stepped out into a major intersection and began to stomp across the street. The man in the sedan who was driving ten miles above the thirty-five-mile-per-hour speed limit told police that this boy had appeared, standing in the middle of the road, directing traffic. Later, bruised and shaken after ten days in the hospital, Daniel explained that he suddenly "woke up" and realized where he was. Frightened, he began running back and forth in the middle of the highway trying to escape, but cars were coming fast in every direction. He stuck out his hand imitating a police officer directing traffic during rush hour, hoping that the sedan suddenly speeding in his direction would recognize his authority, heed his warning—and stop.

DANIEL LOVED THE Catherine Tillotson School and made a great deal of progress there, evidencing no behavioral problems over the course of a month. No one will ever know how Daniel's life would have been changed if he had been permitted to remain at Tillotson or attend another school exclusively for kids with learning disabilities. Unfortunately, his teachers thought Daniel too far gone for help. Perhaps if he had been attended to sooner, or if he had had a more stable home atmosphere, where he could study . . . but such an arrangement was impossible. The Tillotson people theorized that Daniel's IQ might have fallen into the retarded range.

"What does it mean to be retarded?" Daniel asked me.

"It means that your learning disabilities are more serious, and that they are irreversible, meaning that you can't make them much better."

"You mean I'll never read or talk better than I read and talk now?"

"Yes, that's what it could mean, if you were retarded."

"I tried so hard so that staff at Tillotson would like me."

"This had nothing to do with liking you."

"What am I going to do now?"

"What do you think you want to do?"

"I guess I have to try harder."

Daniel's sentiments were encouraging and face-saving, but from that point on, he abandoned the notion of reading and writing. He still wanted to be a policeman, but was willing to settle for a job at McDonald's. It never occurred to him that maybe even a job in a fast-food restaurant would not be possible.

PART THREE

Western Psych

8

MAYVIEW STATE HOSPITAL, about twenty-five miles from Pittsburgh, where both Terri and Daniel have languished, is considered to be
one of the better publicly funded state mental hospitals in the U.S.
Though it has separate units for children, this should not lead anyone to
believe that it is a therapeutic place, according to a former medical
director of the adolescent unit, psychiatrist Scott Waterman.

"How can you disagree?" Waterman asked rhetorically, after stating
that Terri and other Mayview patients complained that they were not
getting good care. "Of course they are not getting good care. They are at
Mayview State Hospital! This isn't a great hospital; the people who work
here aren't the finest of their kind. When Terri told me 'I don't know
what you can do for me here,' I had to admit that I didn't know either."

Waterman refers to "the punitive nature of care at Mayview. At
many hospitals, the staff is nurturing and psychologically minded, but at
Mayview you don't have that. You just have some not-very-well-
educated, not-very-bright people seeing some very disturbed adolescents as bad kids who need to be taught a lesson."

Waterman's criticism is supported by Jacqueline and Kenneth
Harris, whose teenage daughter Maggie was an immediate victim of the
"punitive" regulations—beginning with an intensive "suicide watch."

Maggie had no history of suicide ideation, "but that didn't convince anybody that she wasn't a suicide risk," said Ken Harris. "First they took her teddy bear away—about the only thing in the world that made her feel good—because it had plastic eyes. Then they took her sleeping bag, which had helped her feel warm and safe at night, because it had a zipper.

"Maggie was intensely modest, to the point of terror, frightened about being naked and vulnerable. Sometimes she wouldn't take showers because of paranoia and fear, yet as soon as she was transferred to Mayview, a staff member (men included) was assigned to watch her as she got dressed and undressed, and even when she went to the bathroom. There were no privacy doors on toilet stalls. This was dehumanizing."

"Dehumanizing" may be too strong a description, but "self-protective" and "insensitive" are not. I had received clearances from three succeeding medical directors to visit Terri—and Terri had signed an authorization form permitting me to talk with her and include information about her in my book, but the head nurse continually stonewalled my efforts. Even if I hadn't been writing about her, Terri is a U.S. citizen and has the right to talk with anyone who chooses to venture into Mayview to see her, unless her doctor objects for clinical reasons; I battled the nurse for weeks for such an opportunity.

The privacy forced upon children and families with mental health problems actually enhances stigma and isolation. Locked doors in psychiatric units are reasonable safeguards against "elopement" of patients, but should not exist to keep visitors, who may symbolize the patients' only contact with the outside world, away from people who need them. Forced isolation denies patients their constitutional rights and may enhance their psychosis. Even visitors permitted on the unit were often confined to the kitchen—one cluttered room. Privacy for quiet and dignified talk was denied them. As in many areas of the mental health system in this country, regulations have been established to benefit vulnerable staff and administrators at the expense of the people they have been entrusted to serve.

Once, when Daniel was transferred to a psychiatric ward at a medical hospital, he asked that I bring a camera so that someone could take a photograph of us. He wanted a photo as a symbol of family to put on his bulletin board, but the camera was disallowed because it invaded unit privacy, thus making the institution vulnerable to litigation. It didn't matter that Daniel was lonely and frightened and felt out of place, that the other kids teased him because he could not show them his parents, siblings, pets. It didn't matter that Daniel had given his permission. Even though he had a private room, administrators feared we might unwittingly photograph someone else in the background. Videos and TV showing crime, violence, and sex were allowed, but Instamatics were not.

When Daniel returned to Mayview a couple of years later, I watched helplessly as doctors and nurses systematically tantalized and tortured him with rewards and punishments concerning my various weekend visits. What Daniel wanted most was to go to Pizza Hut or McDonald's—somewhere off the grounds—so that we could share our traditional lunch and conversation. I was his one and only contact with a normal world.

At the beginning of the week on which I planned to visit, he would request and frequently be granted such a privilege, but within a few days it would often be rescinded because of his behavior. Sometimes the behavior was serious, such as threats of suicide and/or aggressive behavior toward fellow patients, such as chair-throwing. I do not condone these actions, but they must be put into context. Daniel had virtually no history of attempting to hurt himself, and his hostility was predictable. His records clearly demonstrated his inability to tolerate explosive incidents in which retarded or seriously mentally handicapped children acted out aggressively. Daniel had always lost his cool during such incidents, as do many victims of PTSD who cannot tolerate threatening and/or highly emotional behavior.

In fact, I would have been surprised if Daniel or anyone else would or could have acted differently under these circumstances. It doesn't take a doctor to realize, based upon his diagnosis and a cursory examination of his history, that Daniel needed to be placed in a settled environment in order to heal and thrive. But he was constantly thrust into an atmosphere in which all the other patients were probably far more seriously ill and certainly more violent and hostile than he. Even the most well-adjusted individuals might become explosive after being incarcerated in close quarters for weeks at a time with people who are profoundly handicapped and out of control. In at least a dozen hospitals and group homes, Daniel lived in the same room or unit with children who were retarded, autistic, incontinent, and unable or unwilling to speak—hardly an atmosphere conducive to the passive behavior expected of him.

And one might legitimately ask: Why punish Daniel in this thoughtless manner for an illness over which he has no control? If victims of AIDS or cancer become hysterical because of the pain of treatment or fear of death, we do not disconnect them from family and friends. Rather, we encourage family and friends to actively participate and urge them to involve patients in activities that will provide pleasure and distraction. How can we justify treating a child or adult who is mentally ill any differently simply because he suffers from an illness of the mind rather than the body?

Private psychiatric hospitals, which have grown from 200 in 1984 to 440 in 1988, are a theoretically viable option to state-controlled institutions, but the quality of care is often uneven. A few for-profit hospital chains, such as the Psychiatric Institutes of America, which operates seventy-three facilities nationwide, have come under attack for over-charging and for forcibly hospitalizing children against their will who are not in need of such intensive treatment.

In a report entitled "Psychiatry for Profit," the *New York Times* interviewed a Palm Beach County, Florida, woman who, as an adolescent, voluntarily admitted herself to one of the company's facilities for anorexia. Instead of being treated for an eating disorder, she was put on antidepressants, causing hallucinations and paranoia. Her insurance ran out after thirty-four days, with $26,000 of charges, including $3.75 per Bufferin tablet, and she was suddenly discharged, her treatment concluded. "One week after I stopped taking medications," she said, "the violence, the fear, and the paranoia disappeared." Charges for private inpatient treatment will easily exceed $30,000 per month. Children and adolescents represent the largest proportion of those under care in private hospitals (41 percent).

The true irony and tragedy, however, may not be how psychiatric hospitals are operated, but whether they should be relied upon to treat our children. The Children's Defense Fund estimates that 40 percent of emotionally disturbed children in the U.S. may be inappropriately hospitalized not only at private institutions, but also at facilities like

Western Psych and Mayview simply because there are no alternatives, even for the most comparatively benign emotional outbursts. Ironically, the consensus among children's mental health experts is that children with emotional problems are best treated in the least restrictive, most normative clinical environment—exactly the opposite of what seems to be occurring.

Theoretically, there are places for children to find counseling and support without having to be hospitalized. Residential Treatment Centers (RTCs) are twenty-four-hour, highly structured facilities that serve children with short-term needs (and offer longer-term care). Few experts debate the potential effectiveness of RTCs as a less expensive and more appropriate alternative to inpatient hospitalization. Nationally, according to the National Mental Health Association, the average cost for treating adolescents and children in a state hospital is $299 per day versus $111.67 for RTCs. If the Children's Defense Fund's estimate is accurate, then an enormous amount of rare mental-health-care dollars is being wasted.

There are other alternatives to hospitalization and RTCs, according to the NMHA. A year of treatment in a day treatment program for seriously emotionally disturbed children will cost $15,000 to $18,000. In experimental programs throughout the U.S., day treatment has prevented the removal of the child from home. For less tenuous situations, intensive in-home crisis counseling might be offered to stabilize the family situation at a six-week cost of $1,100. The "family preservation movement" for kids with mental health problems and their families is gaining momentum and converts among health-care professionals and state and federal health, education, and social service administrators.

In-home crisis counseling or regular day treatment might have been acceptable to Tom and Elizabeth and therapeutic for Meggan Scanlon—if such alternatives had existed. Respite care would have allowed the Scanlons an evening or a weekend to compose themselves. Instead, they were forced to wait until the situation was so intolerable that hospitalization was the only option. Ironically, private and governmental funds are sometimes available on a start-up basis for such programs offering in-home crisis counseling, but despite the proven therapeutic value and the evident cost-effectiveness, neither day treatment nor in-home crisis services are readily available in most areas of the country.

The reason for this outrageously ineffective process can be attributed to how the children are placed—and by whom. Ninety percent of all out-of-state placements surveyed by the NMHA were initiated by state agencies other than mental health authorities, including juvenile justice, child welfare, and education systems, without the input or consultation of mental health professionals. Throughout the U.S., coordination of the mental health and child welfare systems and mental health and juvenile justice systems is rare.

As I have said, under standard operating procedures, one meeting a year is scheduled, about thirty minutes in length, for a gathering of Daniel's teachers, counselors, and supervisors—for educational purposes only. There are no other formal or regular interactions among the people responsible for his future or his life, including his psychiatrist. The only way for Daniel, Terri, or any other kid mired in this system to get people to pay attention and discuss his or her plight is to commit a crime or a self-destructive act. Responsible parties will then rearrange their schedules for emergency meetings, during which time the child's living arrangements or mode of treatment will be altered. Daniel has engineered such crisis situations frequently. Unfortunately, his efforts almost always backfire because there are no options other than increasingly restrictive institutionalization available to him, despite the fact that institutionalization is not often proven to be effective. Virtually the entire mental health system for children and adolescents is based wholly upon institutionalization, and yet, few if any documented studies exist that demonstrate institutionalization is uniformly effective for kids with mental health problems.

Until very recently, there have only been token attempts to significantly revamp the mental health system for children. On the federal level, the most significant initiative is the Child and Adolescent Service System Program (CASSP), established in 1983. CASSP was initially funded at $1.5 million, and has been increased slowly to its current $9 million level, a woefully inadequate figure, but symbolically important. Through CASSP, two thirds of all states have been awarded grants to create programs that would enhance cooperation among the different social service, educational, juvenile justice, and mental health dynasties at the state and local levels. CASSP has also been responsible for inspiring what has been termed the "system of care" approach—agreed upon by a vast majority of the mental health communities as the guiding principles for future care for mentally ill kids.

Initiated by Beth A. Stroul, M.Ed., a consultant to the CASSP Technical Assistance Center at the Georgetown University Development Center, and Robert M. Friedman, Ph.D., of the Florida Mental Health Institute, the system of care is based upon two core values: The first is that the system must be "driven by the needs of the child and his or her family." The second stresses the fundamental importance of community-based care and the establishment of corresponding programs without a heavy reliance upon institutionalization. Stroul and Friedman do not debate the importance of institutionalization for children and adolescents. Many kids with mental health problems need and benefit from the intense therapy, structure, and protection that hospitals and residential treatment centers provide. But not for every child and not all the time; there must be a variety of creative and flexible alternatives, the lack of which is the root of the problem.

At this point, the CASSP system of care provides an essential blueprint for change and has inspired some creative thinking as well as a number of pockets of action throughout the United States. Administrators at the federal and state levels have begun to recognize the problems and have started to make changes, but very little has trickled down to benefit the children and families for whom the goals have been established, and there seems to be no significant change taking place for the immediate future. The people who run the system are slowly changing, but the kids for whom the system has been created remain stuck in time.

9

THE NURSES' STATION on 3 West is located at the front of the unit, separated from the elevator by a set of double security doors. A second set of locked security doors not far from the nurses' station stands at the beginning of a long corridor where boys play football and hockey with balled-up socks or rags. Patients are allotted an hour a day, Monday through Friday, in the small Western Psych gym, enough exercise for the average adult, but just a drop in the bucket for pent-up adolescent males, many of whom suffer from hyperactivity. Weekend and after-school outings are sometimes scheduled at the ball field or a nearby park for hiking and playing, but on any given day, patients receive their most vigorous exercise arguing over who takes the next turn with Nintendo, located in the lounge or day room at the end of the corridor. In addition to Nintendo and TV, there is a pay phone for the patients' use and a couple of sofas, chairs, and tables, mostly serviceable plastic. The unit has fourteen beds in eight bedrooms that open onto the day room.

Activities on 3 West are highly structured, beginning with "wake-up" at approximately 7:00 A.M., breakfast at 8:00 A.M., followed by community meeting at 9:00 A.M.—a time for staff to outline the plan of the day, answer questions, and relieve morning anger and anxiety, if possible. School begins at 9:15 A.M. Grades in the Western Psych classrooms may not be comparable to those earned in public school, although academic credit earned at Western Psych may be transferable.

"Process" groups take place after lunch—discussions focusing on family relations, sexual abuse, and so on—followed by gym time, after which free time is available until dinner. More general group discussions about health issues or personal problem solving might occur after dinner. A big community issue on 3 West deals with the use and care of the limited bathroom facilities, two and a half baths for fourteen boys and girls, a source of constant and heated debate. Three nights a week parents and friends can visit. Before bedtime, some patients attend a relaxation/stress-management group. On 3 West, kids are in their rooms at 10:00 P.M., with radios off by 10:30 P.M.

The routine is considerably more relaxed on weekends, but surprisingly the kids complain about being bored without an array of structured activities. Kids who are depressed don't have the ability to structure time for themselves; they don't know how to find ways to amuse themselves. They isolate themselves, getting agitated and in trouble.

People who knew of my observations at Western Psych would often ask if confining children in close quarters for such long periods of time was necessary. This was a difficult question to answer, for there were different answers at different times for different people. It's true that kids were denied freedom. They could not walk down the street for a Pepsi, play radios loudly, smoke cigarettes, make telephone calls, or ride bikes, all privileges they took for granted at home. This lack of freedom was annoying—even infuriating—a cause of resentment and frustration. On the other hand, most of the kids understood that for one reason or another they needed structure—for protection, if nothing else.

Don Svidergol, thirty-five, who became a psychiatric nurse after working for ten years as a financial analyst for an insurance company, explains that the kids on 3 West "are so dysfunctional that they think a unit on a psychiatric hospital is a normal environment for relationships and friendships." Unless they are blatantly psychotic, his patients refuse to view their peers as sick or emotionally disturbed.

Laure Swearingen, a milieu therapist or MT (nonmedical staff, usually with psychology degrees), describes the patients on 3 West as "kids who have sort of 'run aground.' Developmentally they've stepped off the beaten path. They're like dinosaurs. Within the socially accept-able world, they're extinct." This may be the reason they cling so desperately to one another, long past their discharge.

Many of the patients will not outwardly acknowledge this bond during the length of their admission. They will frequently fight, steal, or compete vigorously for the staff's affection and attention. Only when they are about to separate will the kids display the depth of their feelings of attachment and fear of the future. A message I saw in a "good-bye book," a tradition when discharge is approaching, read: "We did not know each other well, but I pray to God for you. Please pray for me."

ONE WAY TO begin to understand the patient population is to sit in on treatment team conferences, held twice a week for two hours on 3 West, during which time the entire "team"—social workers, physicians, nurses, and MTs—gathers to discuss patient progress over the preceding seven days and subsequently map out a treatment plan for the upcoming week. Because these are usually not life-and-death issues (not in the short run, at any rate), there is less immediacy to the discussions than similar meetings I have attended in a more clinical or "medical" envi-ronment. There is time to joke, to pass the time of day—and to dig more deeply into a patient's inherent problems. I liked this aspect of psychia-try, this sharing of opinions, blending knowledge from different and often opposing points of view.

I am not saying that conflicts do not exist and that everyone's opinions are equally valued. Here, as everywhere else in the medical world, physicians are the kings—they indisputably had the last word on diagnosis and treatment. But whereas in most medical facilities the democratic process is nonexistent, in the psychiatric milieu there is a semblance of give-and-take. This is probably because psychiatry is such an imprecise science: Any psychiatrist who presents his as the last word in diagnosis and treatment is engineering his own humiliation.

The treatment team conference takes place in the playroom on 3 West. We are surrounded by cereal boxes, games, toys, snack wrappers, videos, a scattering of books, and a myriad of mismatched chairs.

Although hospital administrators seem to find adequate conference facilities, doctors and nurses are usually forced to gather in generally uncomfortable and discordant surroundings.

The first patient on the agenda, David, can't seem to control himself, screaming obscenities at any time, day or night. Interestingly, the nurses report that directly after one of those outbursts, he will immediately apologize. So far, no one has been able to determine what is actually wrong with David, thus making effective medication and treatment nearly impossible.

Psychiatrist Viveca ("Vecca") Meyer discussed the possibility of either Tourette's syndrome or attention deficit hyperactivity disorder (ADHD) as David's primary diagnosis. Tourette's syndrome is characterized by motor tics, such as eye-blinking, facial grimacing, and even self-punishment, such as hitting or poking oneself, and/or phonic tics, including obscenities and other rude and inappropriate behaviors. Once thought to be a rare condition, recent epidemiological studies indicate that 1 out of each 1,000 boys and 10,000 girls will suffer from Tourette's, which, like bipolar disease, is genetically mediated.

Children with ADHD will have symptoms that include impulsive, excitable, and even aggressive behavior, lack of patience, inability to concentrate and to remain in one place, temper tantrums, and an overall air of defiance. A few days prior to the treatment team conference, I had accompanied Meyer on her rounds and listened as she questioned David about why he had been sent to Western Psych. "I took a knife," David explained in a quiet and calm manner, "went inside a girl's house, and made her take her clothes off."

"Do you think something like that will happen again?"

"That's the problem. I don't know what I will do and what I won't do." He is tall, lanky, blond, and soft-spoken. Recently, evidence has emerged that David has actually had six different names since he was born fifteen years ago, with each foster parent giving him a different one. "Two years ago, this boy was called Larry Mooney." David has always been overly shy, reluctant to speak. In fact, his first foster placement was with a hearing- and speaking-impaired family because child welfare officials had assumed he could not talk. This "misplacement" was only discovered after the fact at Western Psych when David inadvertently began to move his fingers during a tense therapy session. A social worker recognized the movement as "signing."

Meyer observes that David may also be suffering simultaneously from both Tourette's syndrome and ADHD, as well as obsessive-compulsive disorder (OCD). At the treatment team meeting, Dr. Boris says that he suspects another patient on the unit suffers from OCD. This female patient, aged thirteen, is having trouble following rules. The girl seems absolutely compelled to wash her hands eight times, eight times a day. "That is typical OCD behavior," Dr. Boris says. "The selection of a regular number."

"She's got to check her homework eight times as well," a nurse observes, "and watching TV, she tries to tune into Channel Eight."

There's a new boy in the unit, Joe, who can't seem to stop himself from touching other people. Joe doesn't get the point, despite the many numerous "time-outs" he is penalized. Upon being admitted, Joe experienced great difficulty separating from his mother, and spent the first hour and a half screaming at the top of his lungs in his room. The mother could not remember the occurrence of any psychiatric problem in family members, while the father refused to discuss any relative, especially his mother and father. The staff suspects that the father was both a victim of abuse as a child and a perpetrator of abuse as an adult.

A boy named Steve is so happy on 3 West he doesn't want to leave. "He gets a great deal of attention here, while his mother treats him as if he doesn't exist," says Dr. Boris. "When he was first admitted, he told me that he did not want to go home until he was twelve. When he was told staying that long was impossible, he decided to bargain me down to eight. Right now, he's six."

Steve drew a heart for Boris on a tablet along with a figure representing himself, divided by a line. "Sometimes I love my mother, and sometimes I don't. Sometimes she doesn't play with me, she doesn't talk to me. I don't exist."

The ramifications of a parent neglecting and rejecting offspring are frequently degradation and desperation. Steve and Joe were discovered together in the bathroom the previous weekend, engaging in "an oral-genital contact."

ON ROUNDS AFTER the treatment team meeting, the staff move from room to room, talking with the children.

Eddie, twelve years old, who was sexually abused as a toddler, is writing in his journal. One entry reads, "I do not like to swear at people. I do not like to say I want to jump out of the window. I ate today at the cafeteria. I play frizbe [*sic*] today. I like the teachers fine."

"I want to be Superman when I grow up," he tells his treatment team. "But I look like I'm Harry Henderson."

Anthony, seventeen, is a big, hulking kid with long blond hair and wire-rimmed sunglasses. He loves guns, wants to own dozens of them, but his mother won't permit him to own even one—not anymore. The staff has been attempting to forge a compromise arrangement with his parents in which Anthony could keep one gun at a friend's house and use it only at certain predesignated times and areas. He has previously trashed his house and shot at birds from his bedroom window before his gun was confiscated.

But Anthony rejects the idea. He doesn't want his activities limited. He describes his special maneuver: "I run, dive to the ground, roll as far as I can, jump up, and start to fire full blast. My mother thinks guns are evil. My hobby is raising chickens." Anthony's IQ is 130.

Next comes Ed, seventeen, a "monodelusional patient" who is extremely paranoid and is convinced that everyone he meets is attempting to gas him to death. He is very tall and thin.

Ed is addicted to cigarettes, has a big poster on the wall of his room of a cigarette, smoke curling enticingly from a glowing freshly lit reefer. He has been given Nicorette to chew.

Before being admitted to Western Psych, Ed was knocking on doors and filming unsuspecting people with a video camera. He is mature-looking and has passed himself off as an X-rated film producer. Anytime he sees me, he asks me who I am. When I tell him I am a writer, he says that he is also a writer, composing the story of his own death.

Sally, twelve, says her time on 3 West—two months—is ruining her summer vacation. "I really can't stand it here anymore. These people are driving me crazy."

She's very nervous about an upcoming family meeting, in which her date of discharge will be determined based upon how she and her mother get along. How much longer each kid is required to remain on 3

West is a constant topic of discussion and speculation. It reminds me of the movie *Platoon*, in which soldiers are always counting: "Fifty days and a wake-up—and I'm home."

"But do you feel that you are tolerating your medication?" Dr. Meyer asks Sally. "Do you think it's working well enough for you to go home?"

"Yes," she says.

"Any thoughts about wanting to die?"

"None. They started to go away when I started taking medicine."

"Do you still get upset when kids start to tease you?"

"No, because I ignore them."

"You no longer hear the thoughts and voices that you were hearing before?"

"No."

"Are you worried about hearing those thoughts and voices when you go home?"

"What I'm worrying about," says Sally, "is having a fight with my mother when I go home."

Two days later, Sally's return home was rendered impossible when her mother was admitted to Western Psych.

"Well," Debbie Rubin commented, shrugging her shoulders helplessly after making the announcement at a treatment team conference, "maybe they could share a room."

Ray, twelve, sits and stares, while Meyer tries to engage in a conversation. "Did you talk to your mom last night? How did it go?"

"It went all right."

"Are you worrying about your mom?"

"No." Ray stares and plays with the arms of his chair.

"Do you have any questions?"

"When am I going to go home?"

"That's your favorite question. You do the best you can here, and that's going to help you get home."

"Tell me something," says Meyer. "Are you feeling okay with yourself? Do you have any feelings about wanting to die?"

Ray does not reply.

"No?" Meyer asks. "Will you tell us when you do? Or would you want us to ask you from time to time about these feelings of hurting yourself?"

"Yes," he says. "Ask me."

Dr. Boris asks Jason, ten years old, "How old were you when you started having problems?"

"About eight."

"When did your parents separate?"

"When I was eight."

"Would you like to have your parents back together again?"

"Yeah."

"Do you think that's possible?"

"My dad says it's impossible."

"You think there's a chance?"

"Yeah."

"Do you feel responsible for making your parents break up?"

"I'm trying to get my dad to stop yelling over the phone to my mom when he calls."

"You won't like this," says Dr. Boris, "but I tell you that it is not good for you to continue to deny everything in your life that happens. Yesterday the nurses saw you pushing Larry around. You did it right in front of them, and then you denied it. Now you deny that your parents don't want to come back together. You're afraid to face reality."

Jason shrugs his shoulders and covers his eyes with his arms.

"My visit was good at home," Sanford, fifteen, says as he sits down facing Dr. Boris. "We went outside. I played with my friends. We played torture games. You punch each other in the arms as long and as hard as you can to see how long each person can take it."

Suddenly he stops and looks around. "Where's all that noise in my head coming from? Ohhhhhhh," he says. "Car crash. It's a car crash. I'm dead."

"You never complained of noise in your head before," says Dr. Boris.

"I see a little vision. You know how to focus yourself like a movie projector—all that grain and fog which suddenly becomes a clear picture? That's what happened just now. I was in a car crash. I saw the movie."

"Whose car?"

"My boyfriend's. His name is Carven."

"So you're concerned there's going to be a crash? Do you think it will kill you?"

"Yes," he says.

"Can you predict the future?" says Boris. "Can you read people's minds?"

"Yes."

"Do you think people control your mind?"

"I don't know."

Suddenly Sanford spreads his body across the table and extends his arms. "Ohhhhhh," he says. "I just saw the car crash again."

"How's your mood lately?" says Dr. Boris.

"It's paralyzed."

"Did you say 'paralyzed' or 'paradise'?" says one of the nurses.

"Both," Sanford replies.

Shawn, seventeen years old, is playing with a folding pocket magnifying glass, flipping it with his wrist as if it were a switchblade knife and pointing it menacingly at Dr. Boris.

"Why are you here?" Dr. Boris asks him.

"For fun and experience," he says flippantly. "Now I want to get out, go back to a decent life—parties, school." Dr. Boris begins to ask another question, but Shawn interrupts. "Got a question. Do I get my home visit?" Patients who exhibit good behavior are permitted weekend passes.

"What do you think?" Boris says. "What did I say you had to do to get your home visit?"

"Take my medication."

"And did you take your medication?"

"Bingo," says Shawn. "Can I say something? What are you doing to me? Medication means drugs, and I don't want to be involved with drugs."

"How are you sleeping?" says Dr. Boris.

"Don't take this as an insult," Shawn begins to yell, "but get off my sleeping. I sleep the way I sleep. I do what I want to do. How I sleep is none of your business. How I sleep is exactly how I sleep and that's just about that."

Lisa, sixteen, is a blonde with wire-rimmed glasses. She's wearing a T-shirt and cutoffs. At first she won't talk.

"You look like you really want to cry. Do you feel sad? Are you thinking about hurting yourself? Why do you want to hurt yourself?" Dr. Boris asks. "What about throwing up? Do you feel the impulse?"

"Last night I did, but I controlled it."

"That's good," says Dr. Boris. "It's a good sign. It shows that you care." Dr. Boris tells her about how proud he is of the control she is exhibiting and how she will feel a lot better someday, if she sustains it. "What do you say to that?"

"I say baloney," says Lisa.

"Do you think it's appropriate to vomit two or three times a day?"

"No, but I feel better after I vomit. The food isn't there anymore to make me feel fat."

Dr. Boris says, "I will show you pictures of how the acid from vomiting will ruin the white of your teeth. You will purge yourself of fluid and weaken your heart. Forcing yourself to vomit is very dangerous. What do you want to weigh?" he says.

"I weigh 130, but I want to go to 100."

"What will happen when you go to 100?"

"I'll go to 90," she says. "And then I'll want to go to 80, and then I'll want to go to 70. Anyway that's what you're telling me, but I don't think it's true."

Psychiatrist Kathy Raymer launches into a detailed description of a patient, Alexis, seventeen years old, admitted to 3 West after an incident that began at the youth shelter in which she was living. Directly after a parental visit, Alexis wandered into the middle of a busy street, sat down, and refused to get up. Subsequently, she "cut herself with glass." In the recent past, she has suffered a drug overdose and has threatened to run away, get her father's gun, and blow her own head off. At a court hearing, the judge permitted her to choose between living in a shelter or returning home. Since birth, her father has been physically and emotionally abusive, while her mother has been an ineffective mediator. "Alexis chose shelter care," Raymer comments, "which caused her parents to be angry. Alexis feels like a piece of furniture, moved around from place to place."

Heidi Friend, her teacher on 3 West, interjects that Alexis loves school, talks about finishing high school, perhaps going to college. "But intellectually she is limited with a seventy-five IQ."

Raymer observes that Alexis becomes increasingly upset when her parents either telephone her or come to Western Psych in person to visit—a problem also experienced by Terri.

"Any thoughts or feelings about wanting to kill yourself?" Vecca Meyer had asked Terri during a previous therapy session, which I observed.

"No."

"How did you sleep?"

"Fine."

"Nightmares?"

"Yes." Terri suddenly gets very nervous; her eyes start darting around the room.

"So they began to start up again, those nightmares?"

"Yes, on Wednesday."

"Are they as bad as they were before?"

"Yes," she says.

"Do you have any idea what makes them happen?"

"Yes, whenever I call my father on the telephone, thoughts of killing myself come back."

10

ALTHOUGH THE STAFF maintained a conscious distance from patients, Terri seemed to exert a special grip on the doctors, nurses, and MTs who treated her. MT Laure Swearingen was inherently drawn to Terri, partially because of her dramatic manipulative abilities: "When she needs to win you over, she will put her head on your shoulder or bury her face in your lap. She can make you feel like you're the most important person in the world; ten minutes later, however, she can graphically demonstrate the insurmountable gulf between her life and everyone else in the world."

Swearingen remembers sitting in front of Terri's door after the strangling incident, while Terri was lying in bed bathed in the darkness. "Her eyes were glowing in the shadows. The look on her face was eerie, as if she was staring at a reality that she wasn't experiencing. I was an arm's length from Terri, but I couldn't have reached over and touched her for anything. There was an enormous chasm between us."

As Dr. Boris had explained, Terri was a complicated and dangerous case, representative of all of the problems inherent in the brave new world of child psychiatry. First came the tangled web of dual diagnosis— and what each diagnosis meant and how each impacted and related to the other. It was probably true that she suffered from post–traumatic stress disorder secondary to sexual abuse and neglect.

And she was depressed—but how depressed? What type of depression? "At Mayview she was sometimes weeks in her bed, without moving or talking, curled in a fetal position." To complicate matters, she often became agitated and aggressive, yelling and screaming, pacing constantly, unable to sit down. Her behavior could become so radical—and silly, immature—that it could also be described as manic or hypomanic. So was Terri's diagnosis—or partial diagnosis—"recurrent major depression" or "manic depression"? Dr. Boris believed in the latter, but he wouldn't stake his life on it. If suicide is a clinician's first concern at Western Psych, most nurses and doctors consider the other part of Terri's dual diagnosis, "borderline personality," the most unpredictable and potentially volatile, as evidenced in a poem recited by actress Maureen Stapleton in a video entitled *Borderline Syndrome: A Personality Disorder of Our Time.*

I'm lying here with tears,
Rolling down my face,
I can't seem to keep up
With life's everyday pace.

Life does nothing
But fill me with fear,
I don't understand
Why I was put here.

For life just wasn't
Meant for me.
Because no one really
Cares.

You see.
I have no one.
Not even a close friend.
So now it's time
For my world
To come to an end.

The poem was written by a girl Terri's age, who is discussing how she feels about the way people treat her, especially those whom she most loves. She compares the feeling to being stabbed with a knife, "and everyone who walks by kind of pushes it in a little deeper until you get to the point where you're not going to be able to take it anymore."

Dr. John Gunderson of Harvard University calls "unstable relationships the most discriminating feature of borderline personality," triggered by the inability to judge people with whom they are close, such as parents and/or psychotherapists. Borderline personalities tend to view these people as either all good or all bad, vacillating between the two extremes, which in psychiatric jargon is called "splitting." It's the inability to see a composite picture of another person as having good and bad qualities at the same time.

Dr. Renate Wack of Kirby Forensic Psychiatric Center on Ward's Island in New York explains that "it would be difficult to find borderlines who have good long-term supportive friends." One patient told Wack: "If I feel people start to care then I will reject them before they can reject me. Then somewhere along the line I will get confused and tell them that 'you rejected me.' " Borderlines are also connected to self-mutilating behavior such as wrist-scratching, and recurrent suicidal threats, trademark Terri behaviors.

As I observed Terri on a regular basis, I became concerned about her future. What would happen as time went by? Did she have a chance of recovering? And what did it feel like—inside—what were the gut motivations in mutilating yourself? To understand more about the thoughts and instincts of a lifelong borderline personality, I contacted Gwen V., forty-eight years old. When I first met Gwen, she rolled up her sleeves, revealing a patchwork of stitches, burns, and scars. "My legs are worse," she told me. "I've got them everywhere." Gwen stressed the difficulty of communicating with a borderline personality to whom words do not matter. "No one will listen—unless I cut myself at the same time."

Gwen's psychologist, Irene Pagonis, said that borderlines need to attract attention in unforgettable ways. "I've had patients with cuts which were sutured, who have pulled out the sutures and layered the cuts with feces or mustard. One of the other things we're encountering with borderlines who have been sexually abused is vaginal cutting. Horrible and grotesque, but to them, quite telling."

Dr. Boris once asked Terri if her cutting was painful. "Even when I feel the pain on my skin and flesh, I feel good inside," she replied.

Gwen said that her self-mutilation was often exhilarating. "I want to say, 'Aha! Yes! That's it!' " Gwen's first self-mutilating act occurred in late adolescence. Her younger brother had a crush on a girl who went on vacation for a summer and never answered his letters. "I took a knife and carved this woman's initials into my leg." Later, to demonstrate the extent of her love for a woman, she pressed the hot end of a burning cigarette on her arm. "She saw me burning and screamed, 'What in the hell are you doing?' She grabbed me and we both stared at this huge bubble blistering on my arm. Shortly thereafter, she was out of my life."

Gwen often engineered situations so that people had no choice but to dislike, reject, and disappoint her. Terri duplicates such behavior. In response to her refusal to drink, for example, the nurses will put an IV into her arm. Terri solemnly promises that she will immediately start to drink, as soon as the IV is removed. Three hours later she has refused to drink again. The nurses become angry, to which Terri responds by declaring: "You see! Nobody likes me." This same process is often repeated with her father. She will say something to him over the phone that she knows will make him angry. "He will hang up, and she will say, 'He hates me.' "

Although some medications have been effective in treating borderline personality disorder, intense and consistent psychotherapy is essential to long-term progress. Gunderson refers to success in "the second decade of therapy." Irene Pagonis has been treating Gwen for seven years. Dr. Boris observes that Terri is both very attached to him and angry at his attentiveness and interest. "She is sometimes very nasty. She curses me regularly. Once she threw a chair at me."

Irene Pagonis explained that Gwen has weathered many of her most self-destructive periods, but Terri may expect difficult years ahead. "Borderline personality disorders tend to blossom from about age eighteen to some point in the mid-thirties. Then comes some sort of burn-out. Anger and self-mutilative behavior decreases. But from eighteen years old and onward, 'the fires rage.' "

The confusion over Terri's diagnosis makes the selection of a medication more complicated. Dr. Boris admitted Terri to Western Psych in the summer of 1990 for a series of eight ECT treatments after he had attempted to ease her severe and unpredictable depression, which was exacerbating the symptoms of the borderline part of her diagnosis, through most of the prior year with an array of psychiatric medications. Either the medications Dr. Boris introduced were ineffective or the side effects caused by the medications were too dangerous—or interfered with Terri's ability to function. Dr. Boris was most anxious to introduce an uninterrupted trial of lithium, but Terri, by periodically refusing to eat and drink, did everything in her power to counteract his attempts.

Dr. Boris's decision to try ECT for Terri's manic depression, sending 120 volts of electricity surging through her brain, causing a seizure, symbolized his desperation. Although it is not as controversial as it has been in the past, ECT, considered a last-resort treatment for adults, is hardly ever utilized with children and adolescents because of perceived dangers rather than any real-life threat. The actual fatality rate is only 1 in 25,000 overall, stemming from the anesthesia.

Most opponents are wary of the brain damage ECT is purported to cause, mostly memory loss. Leonard Frank, who underwent thirty-five treatments in 1963 and is currently a leader in the fight against ECT in California, has stated: "My memory for the entire two-year period preceding my last treatment was completely wiped out. My high school and college educations were destroyed." On the other hand, the *British Journal of Psychiatry* published a 1985 postmortem of an elderly patient who received 1,250 ECT treatments revealing no evidence of brain damage.

In fact, many doctors contend that ECT has a better success rate than the "wonder medications" so often touted by psychiatrists in the 1980s and 1990s. The generally accepted cure rate for depression through medication and therapy is 70 percent to 80 percent for severely depressed patients—compared to about 90 percent of the 90,000 people annually who undergo ECT, a process which may also be less costly. A study published in the *American Journal of Psychiatry* demonstrated that patients who received ECT were hospitalized two weeks less than those on medication, generating a savings of $6,400.

Scientists do not understand why seizure cures or modifies symptoms of depression, but ECT was first used therapeutically in Italy in 1938, where seven nurses were needed to protect the patient from convulsions caused by the shock. Today, Brevitol, a fast-acting anesthesia, is dispensed through an IV, while a patient's major muscles have been paralyzed with a muscle relaxant. Oxygen is administered to facilitate breathing. The effects of the electrical charge have been compared to a rocking boat or an automobile ride on a bumpy road, not nearly as severe as dramatized by Ken Kesey in his book *One Flew Over the Cuckoo's Nest*, which showed ECT as violent and destructive. Kesey called the ECT room "the shock shop."

There are two types of ECT: unilateral, in which shock is administered to one side of the brain; and bilateral, in which both sides are targeted simultaneously. Most researchers believe that unilateral ECT will cause less memory loss, while bilateral may be more effective. Some memory loss will occur in either. When I visited Terri soon after ECT she often could not remember having undergone the procedure. ECT will also trigger severe headaches for a few hours, after which some memory will return. Terri's eight unilateral ECTs took place in the summer of 1990, but her immediate improvement was short-lived. Two weeks later, her depression returned, which was why Dr. Boris initiated another six treatments—this time bilateral. When Terri's sullen, hostile, and suicidal mood did not improve, six additional treatments were added the following fall.

Why did Terri seem to improve after each ECT—and why did she feel so happy and secure after the initial ECT trials—and then fall back into a sea of depression? Dr. Boris suspected a "placebo effect"—that Terri responded to the knowledge that she received ECTs and that she was expected to feel better about her life. Reality eventually set in. But on the other hand, if Terri's positive response to ECT was legitimate, then regular maintenance ECT in place of medication might be the answer to her troubles. After her twelve additional ECTs, arrangements could be made for additional treatments regularly, perhaps once a month.

Dr. Boris outlined his goal for Terri, if she is stabilized with ECT. "We want to find a new place for Terri, a group home, where she can form new attachments, to therapists and friends. Ideally this group home would have to be equipped to put in IV units when Terri refuses to eat or when Terri begins to vomit up her food. But first we must make her feel better. We must do everything we can, for this will probably be Terri's last chance."

A few weeks after her return to Western Psych for the final ECT regimen, I went to visit Terri, who invited me into her room. Inside, with the door closed, she began pacing back and forth. She was very excited about Thanksgiving. A nurse from Mayview, Miss Nancy, was taking her home to have dinner and spend the day with Nancy's family.

"Do you like turkey?" I said.

"No, I hate it. I hate stuffing too," she said.

"But you're excited about going?"

Terri had bandages on both arms—one from her IV and the other from a recent scratching episode. "Yes," she said. "I really am."

"When your ECT treatments are over, would you rather go to a group home or a foster home?"

"I'd rather not go anywhere," she told me. "I want to be dead."

She admits that the people on 3 West like her and want to help her—that they're trying—but she indicates her hopelessness with a nonchalant shrug. "Whatever they do . . . nothing will help."

This sense of hopelessness combined with feelings of worthlessness is an oft-repeated theme in Terri's journal, which is filled with metaphoric contradictions. Terri longs to return to her family, even though her mother and father are no longer together, even though her mother's boyfriend has assaulted her and her mother doesn't believe Terri when she tries to report the assaults—or doesn't seem to care. Even though her father has married a woman with radically shifting, constantly confusing responses to Terri's overtures of friendliness. Even though her father, to whom she speaks frequently on the telephone, tells her that she is fat and ugly and that he is going to run away to Canada in order to not have to put up with her anymore. Even though the voices she hears telling her to kill herself most often occur after contact with her family, most often her father.

Those voices inside her head are quite persuasive. At the cafeteria, they tell her to conceal the knife on her tray to use later for cutting her wrists. At school, the voices compel her to palm paper clips and staples to swallow. In her room, they urge her to find things that can be used to

hurt herself—like shoelaces, perfect for strangling. The voices, combined with her father's admonitions concerning her appearance and her
weight, instigate the bingeing and purging that have become part of the
rhythm of her life. She is never safe from the haunting voices of self-
destruction, revealed in her nightmares. She writes:

> I was in my friend's apartment, asleep in one of the rooms.
> Someone breaks into the house and starts to stab me, and all I
> can hear are my screams for help. No one seems to hear me.
> Night time is always the worst for me because that's when the
> sexual abuse usually happened . . .
>
> I had a nightmare last night again. I was walking down the
> street, and this guy with a ski mask on grabs me and takes me
> into this alley and starts to rape me. I was screaming for help,
> but no one could hear me, no one could listen to my cries of
> help. And then he started to hit me with a pipe on the head.
> After he hit me a couple of times, he left me there to bleed. Why
> am I having these dreams? Why me? Life sucks.

The contradictions and confusions are also quite apparent in her
feelings toward Dr. Boris and the staff at Western Psych and Mayview,
where she has spent much of the past few years. On the one hand, she is
desperate to break away from the nurses, doctors, and patients with
whom she has lived for so long and shared her grief and pain. She insists
that she does not want to spend the rest of her life in a mental institution. On the other hand, she understands that these people are her
friends, the only individuals whom she can rely on—and trust.

The day after Thanksgiving she wrote:

> I feel like no one really cares anymore, and I don't know what to
> do. It would be better off if I was DEAD! That's how I feel.
> That's how I feel about going to Ms. Nancy yesterday for
> Thanksgiving. Really got to me because a total stranger took me
> and wants me and my own family don't even want anything to do
> with me. What did I ever do to deserve to be alive? Why do I
> have to be the one with all the problems, the one who spends
> half of her life in mental hospitals, and who no one wants?

I wish I was dead. If I had a way that would work, I would do it, no matter if they tried to stop me. I feel so hopeless, like why should I go on with my life? Why? I feel like nothing is going to get better for me. Everything looks so dark and hopeless . . . I am hearing voices again, telling me that I'm no good, and there's no use for me to live anymore, telling me to choke myself, and keep my knife off the tray and cut my wrists very deep down to the vain [*sic*], and I'm very tempted to listen to it.

I need to talk to someone very bad, but I can't talk or tell them how I'm feeling, it's so hard, especially since I don't trust anyone here. I just wish I could find a way I could succeed in killing myself . . . Why did I have to be born?

The last time I visited Terri on 3 West it was Christmas Eve. Her ECT treatments were over, and in a few days she was to be transferred to an intensive treatment unit for girls called Ridgeview. She was scared, but also very excited. This was the new beginning she had long been waiting for. I said that I would be thinking about her and praying for her, that she was a good person and deserved a happy life. "Do you mean that?" she asked, smiling and giggling.

"Of course I do."

"Well," she replied quietly, "I'm not sure you're right."

11

WHEN FAMILIES OF children on 3 West are available—and willing—Debbie Rubin will meet with them on a weekly basis, first with the parents and, when appropriate, together with the child. Rubin's relationship with the Scanlons is unusually close, not only because Elizabeth and Tom are so candid about their feelings, but also because Meggan has been admitted to Western Psych twice over the past four months. Their sessions have been more than just the fleeting few she might normally arrange with the average parents and/or guardians. Meggan is also honest and articulate, and just as much a veteran of psychotherapy as her parents. With three willing players, discussions will be biting and brutal, but potentially productive. Rubin will not have to devote so much of their time to helping them over intrusive inhibitions.

The first two family therapy sessions I attend with Rubin and the Scanlons are the last two preceding Meggan's second discharge, in December 1990, each lasting about an hour and a half—longer than Rubin's average session, though there is no standard format. Parents can attend with the patient, together or individually, with siblings or other family members, depending upon areas in which problems occur. Because Rubin is attempting to prepare the family for Meggan's return home, she decides to see Elizabeth and Tom for the first part of these sessions and then include Meggan in the second part. Doug has refused to participate.

Meggan had been given a pass home over the Thanksgiving weekend as a transition—a way of helping her integrate back into the regularity of Scanlon family life before being discharged. Elizabeth begins the session optimistically. "We had a good visit with Meggan last weekend." There were no episodes of mania; she exhibited unusual self-control. Over the years, Meggan had acquired the habit of imagining she recognized people across crowded rooms or in other cars driving in opposite lanes, and would attempt to attract their attention, yelling, waving—by any means possible. She was especially friendly and provocative toward motorcycle gangs. But over Thanksgiving Meggan was much more controlled. When Meggan spotted what she thought was a friendly face in a car waiting for a red light, she said calmly, "I think I know those people."

They also visited Winchester Thurston, the private girls' school that Meggan had been attending. Because Meggan was so far behind in her studies, having spent most of the fall term at Western Psych, her teachers were permitting Meggan to drop biology—her most difficult subject—to catch up with other courses.

Elizabeth is appreciative of Winchester's largess, but also apprehensive, based upon Meggan's volatile history. She knows what can happen when Meggan is expected to work on her own. Time without structure and supervision has been detrimental, leading to destructive and embarrassing behavior. Tom and Elizabeth are also concerned about Meggan's free time during the upcoming Christmas vacation. Is Meggan sufficiently different after spending three of the last four months in a psychiatric institution? They discuss the possibility of transferring Meggan to another school with more structure and supervision, but Tom wonders whether the tuition insurance he purchased for three thousand dollars (in case of a permanent suspension) would allow for early withdrawal.

In the video *Four Lives: A Portrait of Manic Depression,* psychiatrist Dr. Michael Schlesser tells a woman named Arty that after forty-two years of suffering approximately eighty manic cycles, she can get well with lithium. Arty is astounded and disbelieving, although it eventually works. Lithium also worked for actress Patty Duke, whose mood swings and erratic and embarrassing behavior nearly ruined her career.

Initially, Meggan had been sent home from Western Psych after an amazing behavioral transformation, attributed to the strict, unyielding structure at Western Psych, along with lithium. But within weeks she was readmitted, her behavior more bizarre and disruptive than at any time before. Then came five more weeks of structured living at Western Psych, with a new regimen of medications—lithium plus Tegratol, an anticonvulsant which has proven valuable in treating manic depression. Once again, Meggan has responded positively. Now she is about to be discharged a second time.

Elizabeth tells Debbie Rubin that after all she and Tom have been through with Meggan she is afraid to be hopeful. She does not want to suffer another disappointment, for she cannot bear to be hurt again. She is concerned about reports from Meggan's teachers at Winchester Thurston that she cannot follow or remember directions. Meggan has always been a good student. If nothing else, Meggan could always apply herself to her studies, especially with a good teacher to inspire and support her. Rubin says that according to her Western Psych teachers, Meggan has trouble with listening comprehension, but is not out of the normal range. Her IQ is the upper average. She is weak in reading words in isolation, but does well in context. As much as they would have liked to pretend that the possibility did not exist, Elizabeth verbalizes what she and Tom are thinking: "Well, I hope it is not the medication."

"It might be the medication," Rubin admits. She is referring to the possibility that lithium or Tegratol could be inhibiting Meggan's concentration.

"I don't want to hear it," Elizabeth says.

"All right." Rubin smiles and shrugs. "It's probably not the medication."

"One step forward," says Elizabeth, shaking her head, "three steps back."

"What do you think about Meggan coming home next week?" Rubin asks.

"I'm really scared," says Tom. "It's like when she was born, and I took her home for the first time, and we were so unprepared. That's how I feel now, unprepared."

"Meggan is like a surgeon who can cut you right where it hurts," says Elizabeth. "For me, it's been nice not having her home. But that's my baggage. I think I have been a failure as a mother."

"You haven't failed," Rubin says softly.

"I feel as if I have no more mother left in me. The mother in me has died."

It is clear from the moment Meggan joins the session that Elizabeth and Meggan have remained constantly in conflict, "jumping down each other's throats," as Debbie Rubin caustically remarks, "at every provocation." Tom is not as combative, but is equally vocal and insistent that Meggan change her behavior. Meggan is tall, with waves of curly light brown hair plunging dramatically over her shoulders. Her hands are also dramatic—and mature. Long graceful fingers, manicured nails, no polish, with silver rings of various designs decorating each of her fingers. Her voice is also quite mature. She could easily be mistaken for a confident college coed rather than the junior high school student she is. At the beginning, Meggan seems friendly and respectful, but at the same time cavalier, as if she were an interested bystander in the proceedings.

The Scanlons tell Rubin that the most important issue to be settled before Meggan's return home concerns her refusal to permit them any privacy—even in their own room and especially after her bedtime. "And changing the actual time of bedtime is not the issue," Elizabeth interjects. "Meggan will agree to most any time, but she never honors her commitments. Meggan goes to bed when she's ready—not a minute before. Sometimes, to have a private, uninterrupted discussion, we sneak down to the laundry."

Tom says to Meggan, "If your return home is going to work out, this issue has to be settled."

Sensing the potential bartering aspect of the relationship, Debbie Rubin asks, "What's in it for Meggan? What can she earn if she's in bed by ten o'clock?"

"Well, she wants more phone hours," says Elizabeth. "But that depends upon her getting her homework done."

Tom says that homework is one issue, bedtime another, but the third issue is that when Meggan decides she wants to do something, she will not take "no" for an answer. Again the discussion takes on familiar, circular patterns, a fact of which everyone is aware. The tension in the room increases, all three Scanlons looking grim.

"If I start arguing with someone," says Meggan, "it's hard for me to stop. It's like having sex and being in heat. You just can't stop no matter how hard you try." Neither Rubin nor Elizabeth blanches at Meggan's honesty. Momentarily piqued, Tom leans back in his chair and turns away. It is no secret that Meggan's mania has led to sexually provocative behavior, but his daughter's candid admission stings just the same.

As the discussion continues, it becomes evident that these are old and tired issues, batted around for years, being debated in front of a new referee and perhaps for slightly higher stakes than before, since Meggan is now older and wants more from her parents, while her parents, more exhausted and frustrated than ever, have become increasingly rigid.

"Well," says Debbie Rubin, "what is it here at Western Psych that has kept you so carefully in control?"

"I have a big goal," says Meggan. "And that is to get out of here as soon as possible."

DR. BORIS JOINS the Scanlons and Debbie Rubin at the discharge meeting the following week. "How do you see Meggan now after these second five weeks at Western Psych?"

"In many ways, I don't think I know her anymore," Elizabeth says. "Perhaps Meggan has become more sensible." Even though Meggan is only fifteen, she has been nagging her parents about being permitted to drive when she comes of age. "But yesterday Meggan admitted that she may not be ready to drive. This is a definite improvement. What is also different is she's not overdoing the 'good Meg' which often occurs after some of our worst confrontations. She becomes sappy and obedient to a sickening degree. So I guess there have been some major changes."

Dr. Boris says that he has tried to teach Meggan "how to treat herself." Not long ago, she confessed that she felt herself becoming hypomanic, meaning that for a distinct period her mood is either elevated, expansive, or irritable to the point where she is unable to exhibit self-control. "That's when prevention must take place." She must inform her parents when she feels it coming—and they must do something about it by applying more structure to keep her in control.

This is not as easy as it sounds. Once Meggan begins to feel hypomanic she will resist any control her parents attempt to enforce. "She's feeling on top of the world, the center of attention. She is not embarrassed about anything. She feels like the leader. So why would she want to put an end to this feeling? It's like an alcoholic person who begins to take alcohol. After their first drink they will go to great lengths not to lose their buzz."

Lithium works very well for 80 percent of Dr. Boris's bipolar patients, more effectively for some than others. It will control the polarity of the moods so that the mania "is not so high and the depression or agitation is not so low." Lithium is most effective in people whose moods are more constant; they are high for a while, then low, then high, with some longevity and regularity. But Meggan's problem is rapid cycling—quick highs, followed by periods of irritability. For these patients, lithium is less effective, unless another medication is added, usually Tegratol.

Lithium can be toxic, but normally not terribly dangerous. "Drinking fluids and urinating a lot is a regular side effect. Meggan must not eat food with low sodium, because less salt means more lithium in the blood which could lead to toxicity. Lithium can also cause a fine tremor, but if she gets more than a tremor or begins to look drunk, immediately call the doctor. Tegratol is dangerous because it can lower white blood cells, so frequent blood tests are advisable. Tegratol may also cause nosebleeds and easy bruising."

Dr. Boris leans forward: "I want you to be aware of the fact that this is not your fault." Although stress in the family can trigger it, bipolar disease is biological. "It's in the genes; it has nothing to do with your actions as a parent. You need not feel guilty."

Elizabeth tells Dr. Boris that her personal therapist thinks that Meggan is not bipolar—that she's really schizophrenic.

"Suppose I have diabetes," Dr. Boris replies. "How do I know I will not have cancer next year? Right now, Meggan is not schizophrenic. How she will look in ten years, I don't know."

After Dr. Boris leaves, Elizabeth says to Debbie Rubin, "We're not a real structured house. I sometimes worry that our household is an inappropriate place for Meggan. We usually take each day by the seat of the pants and see how it develops." Even though lithium and Tegratol seems to be the right combination, Elizabeth insists: "I don't believe in magic. But I am thrilled that the drugs have not negatively affected her. I always resisted medication, fearing that Meggan would be turned into a zombie, sitting there and chewing on her tongue."

Meggan arrives soon after. She kisses her father and whispers something in his ear.

"So are you ready?" says Elizabeth. "Are you nervous about coming home?"

Once again the discussion gets immediately heated about the issue of bedtime. Debbie Rubin interrupts by saying, "How can we give your parents more time together?"

Meggan is not willing to discuss this question. She doesn't like the idea of her parents having time to themselves, explaining that she cannot remember all the things that are important to tell them by 10:00 P.M. "What I hear," Debbie Rubin says, "is that you are uncomfortable about losing access to your parents."

Elizabeth says, "It's the constant interruptions that bother us. I feel as if my time and my space can be violated anytime. That's not fair; it's not right."

"So what are you guys going to do about it?"

Finally, Debbie Rubin says, "Last time when you left the hospital, I was worried about you, but I feel more confident now." Later, Rubin admitted that she was feigning optimism; in her heart she knew that Meggan would be back.

DANIEL

I WILL NEVER forget my first visit to Ward Home. Walking up the front steps and through the double doors, I smelled urine. Water long leaking from the drinking fountain stained the soggy, ragged carpet. A heavyset boy was blocking the doorway, half sleeping, his eyes glassy and dilated. Another boy, tall with stringy, dirty blond hair and pungent body odor, led me to Daniel's room. It was tiny, with a single bed, a plywood armoire, and a metal security trunk. Dirty sheets nailed into the woodwork served as curtains. Music was blasting from every room, the corridors reverberating. Smoke from cigarettes was everywhere; butts, crusts of bread, candy wrappers, and snap tops from soda cans littered the stairways. Upon moving to Ward Home, Daniel had become a heavy smoker. He clutched two packs of cigarettes as we toured the place.

Daniel's learning disability limits his memory. I quiz him regularly about my last name, where I work, what I do; he can never get it straight. We often play this game that begins with Daniel saying, "Ask me a question."

I might respond, "What are the months of the year?" Daniel knows January through August and never forgets December because of Christmas, but he cannot get September, October, and November clear in his mind. Or I might ask, "Where do you live?" He can respond with Ward Home's address and telephone number and Pittsburgh, but cannot fathom Pennsylvania. The concept of fifty states eludes him. But the people who care for him—the social workers with whom he is supposed to bond—are easy to remember because he calls them all by the same name: "Staff." *Staff* took us swimming. *Staff* gave us an allowance. *Staff* made us dinner. Who shaved your head? "Staff!" He had gone outside to play, and crawled into an open sewer line, ending up in a tangle of "jagger" bushes. The "jaggers" had stuck in his hair so staff shaved his head. For months, Daniel looked like a prisoner of war.

Other people in Daniel's life included his child-advocate attorney, Judith Patterson, who represented Daniel in court. Ward Home and Patterson were obligated to take Daniel to Orphan's Court every six months to update a judge on Daniel's case. The judge knew very little about Daniel or the conditions at Ward Home. He never came to visit or asked questions that might flesh out the situation. Daniel was attending school; physically, he was healthy. That was the bottom line to His Honor. The people who were ultimately responsible for Daniel were from Children and Youth Services (CYS) of Allegheny County, the agency contracting with Ward Home for Daniel's care and supervision. From the fall of 1989 to the fall of 1990, three different caseworkers were assigned to Daniel.

I had been appointed Daniel's parental surrogate by his school district, the person who in lieu of parent or guardian approved his Individual Educational Plan (IEP), mandatory for all "special needs" students. I remember once sitting in the lobby of Craig House, Daniel's special school, waiting for a meeting about Daniel to convene. A man in his late twenties walked through the front door and slumped down into a chair. He was wearing an old, wrinkled suit vest with plaid wool pants, a plaid flannel shirt, and a disheveled plaid tie, non-matching. He needed a shave. The sole was flapping from one of his old shoes. I assumed that he was a street person who had come to sleep in the Craig House lobby. But when the meeting was about to convene, the "street person" stood up and I was introduced to Daniel's new CYS caseworker.

Although Daniel was supposed to receive a regular clothing allowance, the money was often not made available until months later. Even then, he was allotted a bare half hour at Hill's Department Store with a generally harried staff to select a wardrobe for the season. Upon his arrival, Ward Home bought him a pair of tan summer-weight moccasins—for the January snow. I have no doubt that Daniel selected these shoes, along with colorful Hawaiian shorts and a couple of bright tank-top shirts, but he did not have gloves or boots the entire winter. From his thirteenth through his fifteenth birthday, he wore running shoes, basketball shoes, aerobic shoes, winter and summer—hand-me-downs from the other kids. Sometimes his shoes were so big the toes flopped, like a clown's.

If the food was not particularly good, it was at least plentiful. He could have as many hot sausage sandwiches, ice cream bars, or Hostess Twinkies for dinner—or lunch, or breakfast—as he liked. He could eat as fast as he wanted. Good manners and good grooming were not priorities, nor was good dental hygiene. Because his teeth had been crooked and uncared for, CYS had arranged for braces. While Daniel was living at his first group home, the braces were tightened as required, once each month. For the next six months at Ward Home, his braces were never tightened and his teeth never cleaned. When I inquired, I was told that the part-time Ward Home nurse, responsible for referrals, had been on maternity leave, so nothing "medical" had been tended to except serious sicknesses and emergencies. Eventually the nurse explained that prior to her leave she had taken Daniel to a dentist who, upon learning that Daniel was on medical assistance, "threw him out of the chair."

Throughout our relationship, Daniel and I have had an ongoing dialogue about fingernails and toenails. Daniel couldn't imagine why his nails grew so fast. His theory was that water made them grow—kind of fertilized his fingers—and since he took four showers a day the length of his nails constantly plagued him. When Daniel was fourteen, I presented him with a fingernail clipper. We sat on the stoop in the front of my house and I showed him how to cut his nails, something he had never been taught. Now, every time I see him, he proudly displays his nails, clean and usually neatly trimmed. "Look, Lee," he will say, beaming, "I remembered."

Daniel always tried hard to please the adults in his life. His constant fear was a future without hope and family. This was especially evident in his ambivalence toward Ward Home. It wasn't as if he was happy with his surroundings, but it was his only home; the staff were his only family.

No one actually realized the importance of this attachment until the day he was officially "terminated" because he had started a fire that destroyed his room and endangered the lives and property of everyone living in the facility.

At first, Daniel was thought to be a hero for discovering the fire and saving his roommate's life, but the staff soon concluded that Daniel had actually been responsible for the fire. Despite warnings not to touch an old, faulty space heater, Daniel had surreptitiously taken it from a storage area, set it close to his bed, and gone to sleep. Daniel's excuse was that it was winter, the radiator in his room didn't work, and he was cold. Staff admitted that the room had no heat, but blamed Daniel for persistently toying with the valve that operated the radiator—until he broke it. At any rate, the fire started, destroying the furniture and most of his and his roommate's possessions, and when the smoke, soot, and confusion cleared, Daniel was confronted by staff who told him that his residence at Ward Home was "history."

Daniel's immediate reaction was muted. He and Terri and other regularly institutionalized kids expect rejection and disappointment, constantly attempting to pretend that no one—especially an adult—can ever hurt them. But Daniel soon became agitated. He told staff that life was no longer worth living, that his birth was an unfortunate accident, that no one had ever wanted him, especially his mother, and that now that he was being thrown into the streets (this was not true; a transfer would be arranged), he was planning to do away with himself.

Daniel had been meeting regularly with psychiatrist Janice Forrester, who initially had been instrumental in extricating him from Mayview, but she was out of town. A psychologist taking her calls, familiar with Daniel's case, interviewed him at the request of Ward Home. Daniel's ideation—his plan for suicide, hurling himself from a nearby bridge—was sufficiently specific, justifying involuntary commitment. Daniel was admitted to a private nonprofit psychiatric hospital, Allegheny Neuropsychiatric Institute (ANI) for nearly a month—at an approximate cost of $25,000.

Later, to complicate matters and further exacerbate Daniel's feelings of isolation, Dr. Forrester left as medical director of the ANI unit to which Daniel had been admitted. When I went to see Daniel with the Pizza Hut pizza and Pepsi we always shared, he was heavily medicated, but understandably stunned. "Everyone leaves me," he said. "I'm so afraid that one day I will be thrown out into the streets. No one will help me. I'll be living in a cardboard box." He began to cry.

"That will never happen to you, Dan. I can't conceive of it," I lied.

"Then I really would kill myself," Daniel said. "Even now I think my life is over. What's my reason for living?"

PART FOUR

Family Therapy

❧

12

YOU WAIT FOR Dr. Kenneth Stanko in a wilderness of neutrality: beige carpet, beige bench chairs with matching beige baseboard, beige wallpaper with large but unobtrusive diamond designs, a decorative wall plaque in a marbled pattern—also beige. A fan, blades moving at a restful speed, hangs from a cream-colored ceiling; classical music oozes from two brown speakers hanging high on the wall. As part of a diffused lighting arrangement, there is a side table, covered with Plexiglas, with a built-in light emanating a soft fluorescence.

Although our appointment is for 10:00 A.M., and it is now fifteen minutes past the hour, I do not knock on Stanko's door or peek through his keyhole. Anyone who has been in therapy knows that a session begins with patients cooling their heels in the psychiatrist's anteroom, wondering if they have been stood up. Some psychiatrists will signal your turn by opening the door, while others will open the door, catch your eye, and crook a finger. Stanko will actually come out and greet you, flashing a big smile and pumping your arm with warmth. Stanko is tall and slender, with a long pointed nose, a pointed chin, and large tortoiseshell glasses that envelop his narrow face.

The tone of the decor continues in his inner sanctum: The industrial carpet and three well-worn easy chairs, arranged in a triangle, are beige.

In addition to his highly polished maple desk and a tiny battered bench on which kids might sit or play, there are a brass table lamp, a brass floor lamp, and a porcelain urn desk lamp.

Stanko's eyes are very expressive, as are his hands, frequently in motion when he talks. When he is being especially intense, he points and pokes the air. He holds his hands up, raises his palms, and spreads his fingers in a fanlike semicircle, then twists his wrists back and forth, as if he is screwing a light bulb in and out of its socket. He has a large mouth with which he can create masks of dozens of moods—from exhilaration to depression—while describing interactions between himself and his patients. He shrugs a lot and will whisper or raise his voice for emphasis. He tends to act out answers to my questions on occasion, providing both sides of a representative dialogue between patients and their therapists.

I first began meeting with Dr. Stanko because I was interested in learning more about how psychiatrists in private practice function—how their work compares to the psychiatry I had been observing in institutions such as Western Psych. What kind of people were these men and women behind their psychiatric facade? Were they as bright, dedicated, and sensitive as they would have their patients believe? Or did the banal caricatures of psychiatrists in movies and books contain more than an element of truth? Even many physicians believe the worst about their psychiatric colleagues.

Usually, Dr. Stanko will hang his perfectly pressed blue suit jacket in the closet, walk across the room, and settle into his chair. Despite a full day and evening of appointments, his oxford cloth shirts always seem unwrinkled and his fashionable, tasteful ties remain neatly knotted at the neck. His wife, Anne Muscarella, has told me that her husband has "a great appreciation for all-cotton shirts, and he especially enjoys selecting his ties at Saks Fifth Avenue." Stanko is also an avid bird-watcher. At home, binoculars hang on a hook by the back door, overlooking a patch of woods behind a spacious grassy yard.

Even though he left the seminary in northwestern Pennsylvania after only two years, Stanko appreciated the isolated and protective lifestyle it offered, which is why he enjoys being alone in his office or working with people in close quarters for such long stretches. He entered the seminary for the wrong reasons, however. "I had not developed physically and/or socially as fast as my peers. As the smallest and skinniest kid in class, I was anxious about my self-image. So the seminary was safe, although I soon realized I had no interest in leading a monastic and celibate life."

Normally, our discussions were unplanned and open-ended. Stanko pontificated, complained, informed, and observed spontaneously. I nodded, asked questions from time to time, took notes. Each of our sessions was tape-recorded, a process of which Stanko was quite solicitous, always waiting patiently until I unzipped my briefcase and placed the tiny black device on the table beside my chair. This was usually the signal to begin.

Our meetings were initiated for purely informational purposes, six months before I had ever heard of Tom, Elizabeth, and Meggan Scanlon. I had imagined that if our relationship developed, I might try to convince Stanko to allow me to meet one of his patients and obtain permission to sit in on a few sessions. When I met the Scanlons and began interviewing them, I had no reason to believe that they would become Ken Stanko's patients after Meggan's second discharge from Western Psych.

Stanko had been recommended by one of Elizabeth Scanlon's contacts in a support group for parents of kids with mental health problems she and Tom were attending. Stanko had initially refused when Elizabeth contacted him because he was overcommitted, but she was characteristically persistent. "What do you mean, you're too busy?" she had asked him. "We need you."

Stanko relented. He met with the Scanlons for an evaluative session two weeks before Christmas 1990, soon after their final "discharge" meeting with Debbie Rubin at Western Psych, but his real work with Meggan, Tom, and Elizabeth began early in January.

THE ATMOSPHERE IS combative from the very moment the door is closed, the warring factions seated and the amenities dispensed with. The quiet feeling of peacefulness and unity with which Debbie Rubin had attempted to end their last meeting had not been sustained twenty-four hours after Meggan returned home. Stanko suddenly found himself in the heat of an ongoing firefight among people he did not know, about issues of which he was not completely aware—a tense and volatile situation he was expected to resolve with intelligence, style, and undue haste. It was an overwhelming task. The relationship between the Scanlon family and Kenneth Stanko seemed to rarely achieve an acceptably steady foundation.

Meggan's driving was the critical subject of debate for this first session, a topic that always provoked Elizabeth, who pointed out that whenever Meggan fixed her mind on something, she would beat the subject to death until she got her way. "Her sixteenth birthday is five months away, and at eleven o'clock, when we are ready for sleep, she wants to talk about driving. I don't mind talking about her driver's license; the discussion isn't forbidden. I'll be happy to debate. But give me a break—a night's sleep. Let's pick it up in the morning." She slapped her fist into the palm of her hand. "But not Meg. No way!"

Stanko nodded, staring in a concerned manner toward Elizabeth, as psychiatrists will do. He was about to comment, but Elizabeth immediately changed the subject. "I got a phone call from a teacher [at Winchester Thurston] yesterday. Meggan is sleeping in class."

"It was not actually in class," Meggan objects. "In the lounge and in the gym. It wasn't during class."

Sleeping in class or at school is new, Elizabeth observes. Meggan's sleeping problems have been centered at home. "We want Meggan to be asleep by ten o'clock—not just starting her homework. But I might as well be talking to a balloon, because she doesn't listen. After school and dinner, she talks on the telephone, fights with Doug, harps on us. And then suddenly it's bedtime—and she hasn't started homework. No wonder she is sleeping in school; she stays up all night."

Once again, Stanko stares, scribbles notes onto a pad and nods, but once again Elizabeth redirects the discussion. "We said to Debbie Rubin when we brought Meg home that we would have to get to know her again, but we now realize that we really know her only too well. She is just as oppositional as before. Meggan won't even take her medication at the right time. We plead and beg. Whenever we tell her to take it, she replies, 'When I am good and ready.' "

"We looked at lithium as our lifesaver," Tom interjects. "But Meggan has turned the medications into a club to beat us to death. I find myself following her all over the house like a little kid, saying 'Did you take your medication?' " He shakes his head and shrugs his shoulders. "I'm sick and defeated already, and it has only been three weeks since Western Psych."

Stanko leans back in his chair, employing his hands as a headrest. He explains that lithium remains in the bloodstream for only short amounts of time and that when a daily dosage is missed, the effects of the drug are minimized. Another twenty-four hours are required for it to be reintroduced. Because Meggan is scheduled for twice a day, missing one dose is not terrible; she can take both pills later without harmful effects. And Tegratol, her other medication, is ingested only once a day. "So it is not a disaster if Meggan refuses or forgets. In fact, whether or not she takes her medications is her problem—not yours." This is the first hint of the treatment plan Stanko is going to introduce.

Dr. Stanko explains that Meggan should be permitted to resolve certain issues on her own, including when or whether she takes her medications. "Your role is to share your thoughts and to establish acceptable boundaries in your own house. But back off and give Meggan leeway to make her own decisions and seal her own fate." At this point, Stanko requests that Tom and Elizabeth leave the room.

Once alone with Meggan, Stanko clarifies that the confidentiality of their discussions will remain sacred. "Is there something you want to tell me that your parents don't know about?"

Meggan says that her parents do not understand how teenagers really act and that she realizes her parents are afraid she will become sexually active again. But such behavior won't be a problem because Meggan feels she has it under control.

Stanko is impressed with Meggan's resolve. To most of her comments, he responds, "I hear you, Meggan, I hear you." He tells Meggan his plan: From this moment forward, he should be utilized as the family mediator for any serious conflict, thus theoretically eliminating the need for Meggan and her parents to argue. "Any problems are to be put in my lap. Call me on the telephone or save them until our next meeting." He repeats his plan of action to Tom and Elizabeth when they are invited back into the Stanko inner sanctum. "Whatever your concerns—her mood, her sleep, medication—you can call me, and I will get back and tell you what you need to know."

As the session ends, Tom and Elizabeth are agreeable, outwardly.

Privately, they are dubious because, for one thing, Meggan does not have the patience to wait for a telephone mediator to aid the decision-making process. She expects her demands to be satisfied on the spot, despite the difficulty it may cause anyone else involved. Nor do they mention—or perhaps they don't even realize—that neither of them is temperamentally suited for such a laissez-faire philosophy. But they are willing to try anything, and so they vow to lock the door to their bedroom. "If Meggan stays up late and falls asleep in class, it is her problem—so long as it doesn't interfere with anyone else in the family," Elizabeth promises.

For this and all subsequent sessions, Stanko remained seated at his desk while the Scanlons situated themselves in the beige easy chairs. I sat at the opposite end of Stanko's desk, closest to the window. I could look down from the second floor and view the snow-encrusted landscape of Stanko's office complex and the circular drive with a scattering of reserved parking spaces for special tenants. At the front of the building, a fashionable restaurant with a comfortable outdoor cafe was being renovated. It occurred to me repeatedly, each Wednesday afternoon that we met, that this pleasant and traditional setting was completely inappropriate for such prolonged pain and frustration.

A WEEK LATER, the atmosphere the Scanlons bring into Stanko's office is grim, rather than volatile. Meggan's hair is disheveled and her complexion seems gray and pasty. Dark circles have been etched under Tom's and Elizabeth's eyes. Tom stares at the carpet and shakes his foot, while Elizabeth seems icily removed.

Meggan begins. After having battled with her mother most of the weekend about the now familiar subject, driving, or more specifically in this case, car insurance, Meggan and Elizabeth have agreed to no longer communicate, not only about driving, but any subject whatsoever. This silent state of war remains in effect as long as the Scanlons are in therapy with Stanko.

Tom, constantly walking a narrow and dangerous tightrope between daughter and wife, is sympathetic to Meggan, assuring her that when the time comes, he will subsidize her insurance. Meggan either doesn't believe her father or cannot process the information. She launches into a rambling plan about getting a job cleaning houses. She tells Stanko in minute detail how she will find customers, charge for services, and spend her profits. Meggan is an obsessive housecleaner, her parents explain—without any consideration for other people's privacy. "If Meggan wants to vacuum at midnight, she'll do it," Tom says.

"Isn't this a violation of normal boundaries?" Stanko asks. "Meggan's obsession to clean should not interfere with the entire family's sleep."

"With Meggan, it is often easier to give in than to suffer the trauma of a fight." Tom admits that this is how Meggan bludgeons them into compliance. "But . . ." He shrugs helplessly and lapses into a morose silence.

Meggan, nearly in tears, says that she has joined a study group at Winchester Thurston, but her parents refuse to recognize her positive efforts. "I try so hard to please my parents, not to get in their way, to help them as much as I can and to do better with my grades. My mother doesn't believe that I am even trying."

As I sit by the window scribbling my notes (no tape recorders for these sessions), I wonder whether to believe Meggan. She is obviously distraught, but is she acting—or are her feelings genuine? The Scanlons contend that Meggan's performances in front of adults, especially strangers, are of Academy Award quality. Stanko has said that bipolars believe wholeheartedly in themselves during their most manic periods. Meggan may not be telling the truth, but it would also be inappropriate to say she is lying.

After asking Tom and Elizabeth to leave the room for a few minutes, Stanko turns to Meggan: "Tell me about your boyfriend."

Meggan discusses their courtship. They've seen each other twice since 3 West. On Christmas Day, she went to his house, and on New Year's Day, they took in a movie. He has proposed marriage, and she is wearing his engagement bracelet. Meggan vacillates between total commitment or keeping herself open for somebody else, but she also misses him. "I cry in school all the time. Like now," she says, tears streaming down her face. Meggan laughs when Stanko asks what she would do if she got pregnant. "I have no intention of getting pregnant. My parents would blow balloons in their brains if I did." Stanko asks how many times during the day she actually cries about John. In school, at home, and then she cries herself to sleep, Meggan says.

"Most of the time during school I am manicky and hyper. I'm not sexual, but I am very interested in sex. I find myself jumping on people."

"Literally?"

"Yes. In biology class, I cracked a joke about sex, and I yelled things out without thinking."

"When you yell these things out, do you think they are funny?"

"No, it's embarrassing. But I can't help it." She pauses to run a hand through her hair and then shakes her curls back from her shoulders. "I've also been telling strangers my life history. People I hardly know. I wish I could stop," she tells Stanko earnestly. "I'm also talking too fast, and talking too loud. When I'm talking loud I know in my heart I am trying to prove something to somebody else."

"What's that? What are you trying to prove?"

"That I am better—or just as good as anyone else."

Stanko is listening carefully, nodding often, bolstering her confidence by saying, "Meggan, I understand completely!"

She is very disturbed with her parents' refusal to treat her with understanding and respect. At one particularly heated moment earlier this week, her father threatened to send her back to Western Psych.

"I told him 'You can't send me back to the hospital.'"

" 'Want to bet? Pack your bags.'"

"I told my mother we should discuss our problems with Dr. Stanko, and she told me, 'I'm not talking to him anymore.' " Stanko raises his eyebrows, but does not respond.

When the parents are asked to return, Elizabeth is angrier than ever, ready to explode. She repeats that her daughter is obsessing about automobile issues, and that Meggan has also found a way of utilizing Stanko's treatment plan as a wedge for her own purposes. "I told Meggan to go to her room, and she said, 'You can't tell me to go to my room, you have to ask Dr. Stanko.' "

The session lasts a lot longer than the fifty minutes Stanko has reserved. Because other patients are waiting, and nothing between the Scanlons has been resolved, everyone—patients and doctor alike—is edgy and morose. After they leave, Stanko sinks into his chair and presses his palm to his forehead for thirty seconds of meditation before calling his answering service to check his telephone messages. He returns a phone call to an attorney for whom he is consulting, then stands up and opens the door to the anteroom, where he greets his next patient with a broad, welcoming smile and ushers him in.

13

A FEW DAYS LATER, I met with Elizabeth Scanlon for a brown bag lunch in my office at the university, where we talked for two hours about life with Meggan and the latest crisis their daughter had precipitated.

"Saturday night, we were playing pinochle. We had given Douglas permission to go roller-skating until midnight. Meggan was home alone when she finally decided that she would drive the family car." The roads were icy and slippery—the weather had been blustery all day—but Meggan started the car, backed it out. Halfway up the driveway, she lost control and bounced over a curb that separated the driveway from a sloping yard. Suddenly the car was stuck, hanging precariously over an embankment.

At first Meggan panicked. She phoned a neighbor, swore him to secrecy, and begged him to come to her aid. Knowing Meggan, and figuring that the car was safest right where it was—inoperable—he declined, advising her to go back into the house and wait for her father to come home. But Meggan wasn't to be deterred. She returned to the car, started it, threw it into first gear, floored the accelerator, and popped the clutch. Somehow, ingeniously and luckily, she managed to dislodge the vehicle, get it back onto solid ground and into the garage.

The average fifteen-year-old might learn a lesson from this experience, having gotten herself out of such an embarrassing and vulnerable dilemma. Meggan, swelled with confidence, soon returned to the scene of the crime, started the car, and resumed her adventure. This time, she successfully navigated the narrow drive, then conducted a slow and deliberate tour of the neighborhood, as if she had been driving for half her life—rather than just half an hour.

Confidence and the weather got the best of her when she returned home. Losing control in the snow, she slid down the driveway and smashed into the garage door. The damage was easily discovered by Tom and Elizabeth when they arrived home, but Meggan chose to remain silent, while her parents decided to wait to see how long it would take her to come clean.

Sunday, as Tom drove Meggan to the library for a meeting of her study group, he said, "You know, sometimes things happen that you are reluctant to talk about. It is really important, especially when your family is concerned, that you discuss those things. We would understand." Meggan was silent at the time, but when he picked her up later in the afternoon, she related her Saturday-night adventure.

This was not a confession, and Meggan was in no way contrite, Elizabeth stressed. She was proud of the incident, even though it had resulted in damage and had seriously endangered her life. " 'Guess what, Dad!' " Elizabeth mocked her daughter. " 'I had the car out. Spun it around the neighborhood, and it was great. I'm great. But I am not sorry. What's the point of being sorry? What does that accomplish?' "

As I looked at my notes later in the day, I thought that Meggan had actually responded to her father's veiled request to tell the truth about driving the car in a reasonably acceptable manner, considering Dr. Stanko's recommendations concerning more compromising behaviors from both factions. Tom too had acted appropriately by not pressuring Meggan to bare her soul; he had introduced the topic in a subtle manner. After a few hours of reflection, Meggan had confessed in a way she perhaps needed to protect her own dignity and self-image. The results were unsatisfying to Tom, Elizabeth, and probably also Meggan, but at least the subject had been broached and discussed. Combat had been avoided. And Meggan admitted that technically she had committed an illegal act—and that she deserved to be disciplined. Whether she was willing to accept the discipline when and if it was imposed was another matter. But some headway had been made. Perhaps Elizabeth might have agreed with my objective analysis if she had been able to be as dispassionate as I, but fifteen years of conflict with her daughter had diminished her capacity for compromise and skewed her orientation toward the situation.

As she was wont to do, Elizabeth became obsessed with all of the ways in which Meggan was failing. Or, to put it another way, Elizabeth could not stop talking about how Meggan continued to sap energy from her parents and drag down the entire family. From the story about Meggan stealing the car, Elizabeth launched into the story about Meggan's trials and tribulations at school.

"Meggan does seem to be trying to study," said Elizabeth, "but something is haywire. She had a biology test the other day, and when she came home she said, 'I think I got a B.'" Meggan discovered the following day that she earned a $D-$.

"I said, 'Where do you think you went wrong?'"

"She said, 'Well, I lost all the points on the essay. And there's going to be essays on my tests next week. What am I going to do?'"

"I said, 'Okay, for an essay question read the question and think of three to five key points that are important. Then write an opening-line sentence. Get your thoughts going and do a closing sentence. And that's your answer. Do you think you can do that?'"

"'Yeah, I can do that.'"

"It's like nobody ever told her how to write an essay. I know her teachers have gone over those simple points a hundred times. Anyway, I looked at her answer when she got the paper back. She wrote one sentence and drew two pictures. The teacher wrote, 'Cute picture; wrong concept.'"

Elizabeth told me that she and Tom were seriously thinking about removing Meggan from the house, but convincing Meggan to leave home without having a horrible fight might be impossible.

"In times past, I could drop her off in any setting with a bunch of kids or another parent and she never gave us headaches. But since North Country and Western Psych, there's been a complete about-face. I have recently tried to talk with her about Girl Scout camp, but she has said repeatedly, 'You can't pry me out of this house.' My nightmare is that we're going to have to drag her out, literally kicking and screaming.

"I've heard of parents taking their kids in the car and saying, 'We're going to go visit an aunt in Philadelphia,' and guess where they are really going? Some institution somewhere, with the truck behind them that the brother-in-law is driving with the child's clothes and possessions.

"Oh, God." Elizabeth began to cry. "I don't know if I have that kind of energy—or courage. You have to be completely desperate to do something like that. Those are feelings I don't even want to touch. Everybody has had a heartache in life, but you don't realize what it feels like to want to murder your own kid. Meggan is strangling us to death."

MEGGAN IS SO deeply involved in her study group that she cannot possibly attend the regular session with Kenneth Stanko this week. This is just as well, for the Scanlons' time alone with Stanko would provide the perfect opportunity to discuss their desire to remove Meggan from the house. But they abandon their agenda as soon as the meeting starts, allowing their obsession to talk about how Meggan has sabotaged their lives to overwhelm them. Repeatedly, they experience great difficulty telling a story from beginning to end or making a point without digressing on rambling tangents.

Elizabeth describes Meggan's "honeymoon periods." First, Meggan will do something oppositional and obnoxious. A terrible battle ensues. Sometimes she wins, sometimes she loses, but as soon as the issue is resolved, a period of perfection will follow, with Meggan sweet as pie. "And then, as soon as we think Meggan is really changing, has finally turned the corner and become a decent human being, she will do something terrible, launch into a day-long tantrum—whatever."

"She terrorizes us," says Tom flatly.

"If she doesn't get what she wants," says Elizabeth, "she puts up such a fuss that we have no choice but to give in." She raises her voice and leans forward: " 'You want a ride to Tokyo, Meggan?' " Elizabeth mimics herself. " 'Okay, get in the car.' " Tom tells a long story about fixing a spaghetti dinner one evening. Meggan walked into the kitchen and announced that she didn't want spaghetti. In fact, she didn't want dinner. So Tom served Douglas and they enjoyed a pleasant dinner conversation. They were doing the dishes when Meggan returned. "Now make me my spaghetti," she demanded, pointing at her father as if he were a servant. "Do it now."

"I wanted to say, 'I'd sooner live on Mars than fix you spaghetti,'" said Tom. "But I knew what would happen if I refused. We would have had a destructive battle. Doug would have been made crazy. So," he said, pausing to lower his voice and chuckling at his own helplessness, "I made her spaghetti and kept my mouth shut."

"What would have happened if you had not fixed the dinner?" Stanko asks.

"She would have gone on and on—talking, yelling, demonstrating. Telling stories about how cruelly we treat her to friends and neighbors— anyone she might telephone who would listen. It never ends."

Stanko interrupts. "I hear you clearly," he says, raising his palms. "But let's move on." He is attempting to redirect the conversation to ways of countering Meggan's oppositional behavior, but the Scanlons cannot stop dredging up the ways in which Meggan controls and frustrates them.

"She is a master of these cute little flicks of the verbal sword," Elizabeth interjects. "She is always saying things that hurt me."

"Manics," says Stanko, "are incredibly intuitive."

"Sandy," says Elizabeth, referring to her own therapist, "says that it is actually 'random selection.' Meggan probes and pushes in every conceivable direction until she discovers my most vulnerable areas. She attacks repeatedly until she hits a target—any target."

Elizabeth looks up and raises her eyebrows in reflection. "Meggan will often tell me, 'You will always love me, no matter what I do to you,' and I always reply, 'No, I won't.' But we are actually both right. I will always love her, but at the same time, I will never love her again."

"What we have been praying for is that Meggan will turn into a human being somewhere between the ages of twenty and thirty. But during the past few weeks we have come to realize that we will never be able to wait that long," says Tom, finally inching his way toward the subject that they had intended to broach.

"Some parents have been known to set kids up in apartments when they are seventeen," Stanko says. He is actually joking, attempting to relieve the tension, but neither Tom nor Elizabeth is smiling, perhaps because they are seriously pondering his suggestion.

"Okay, let's talk about Meggan and how we will get through life until she is twenty," says Stanko.

"Eighteen," says Elizabeth, "no longer."

"It's important for you to understand," says Stanko, "that this behavior with Meggan is going to continue. Our treatment might make her better, but we are not going to turn her into another person."

"Why not?" says Tom. "What a great idea!"

Suddenly, Tom and Elizabeth look at each other and burst out laughing. During all of the many months I observed the Scanlons, I most admired their ability to laugh at a time when their future looked particularly bleak. Tom and Elizabeth, and sometimes even Meggan, were able to view the tragedy of their situation with a rare humor that helped them survive.

Stanko waits for the laughter to subside. He tells the Scanlons that they must reorient their thinking and become more realistic. They must accept the fact that Meggan will not be easily controlled in the short run, while remaining optimistic about the future. The immediate challenge is for them to learn to respond more effectively to Meggan's behavior. "You can't be oppositional to someone who is oppositional," he tells them. "It's like banging your head against a brick wall. You will only hurt yourselves."

"But when we ignore her," says Elizabeth, "she escalates. The last time we ignored her she sat on a windowsill, threatening to jump. We called Western Psych and they told us to call the police and have her arrested. We are not unfamiliar with the things you're telling us to do. We have tried many strategies. Basically, she stands there with her chin sticking out and dares us, as if to say, 'Okay, you sons-of-bitches. I'm ready for anything. Just try to get me.'"

Now the subject of extricating Meggan from the Scanlon milieu is finally upon them. Elizabeth approaches with a rush. "We've tried to be nice; we've tried to be calm. I've stood on my head, but I tell you, Dr. Stanko, I'm exhausted. Okay, I understand that she's never going to be better. But what I want to know from you is, can anybody help her?" Elizabeth leans forward and her voice changes to a tone of tearful, pleading desperation: "Can anyone, anywhere, help my child?"

Elizabeth's sudden emotional appeal seems to catch Stanko by surprise. He stares at Tom and Elizabeth, not knowing exactly what to say. When he does begin to speak, he avoids acknowledging their pain and desperation, attempting to stabilize the situation by discussing the importance of maintaining treatment—medications and talk therapy—despite the difficulties.

"Isn't there any place more structured to send her for help?" Elizabeth asks. "At least when she went to Western Psych, they managed her. And it was a welcome vacation for us."

Tom asks Stanko how much he expects them to bend to Meggan's demands—then goes off on a tangent once again. "Tonight, for example, we will be ready to go home at six o'clock but she will not be ready to go home from the study group until seven o'clock. Now what do I do? Wait for her till seven o'clock? Or do I go home for a half an hour and then return and pick her up? Or do I let her fend for herself?"

"Let the chips fall where they may," Stanko replies. "Reason with her. Say to her that you will cooperate this time, and this time only. No more after that. She must bend, if you bend." He continues to provide examples of rational reactions in response to Meggan's irrational behaviors, while the Scanlons sit and stare, numb, dumbfounded, and beaten. They do not want to hear the same old message. They want a cure—or an escape. Elizabeth asks again, pleadingly: "Is there another place that Meggan can go to?"

With a sigh and a defeated shrug of his shoulders, Stanko tells them about therapeutic boarding schools. "But they are ridiculously expensive and will only work if Meggan wants them to." If they continue to establish limits and to compromise, just maintain the status quo and not let it get any worse, the results will probably be the same "as if she went to boarding school and you spent all that money," an estimated $50,000 per year.

"What about us then?" says Tom. "What about sacrificing the lives of three people for the sake of one?"

Stanko nods, as if he understands exactly what they are saying. But once again, he only repeats the concept of avoiding direct opposition at all costs.

Tom and Elizabeth are numb and crestfallen. This was their last hope, their one chance to escape, and their psychiatrist has now eliminated that option. Tom's eyes are closed and his chin is resting in his palm. They talk a little about the medication. Should they try more Tegratol? Should lithium be eliminated? They report that the Clonipine Stanko has prescribed is helping Meggan sleep at night, making her calmer. The discussion, which began with passion and fire, is now cold and wooden in tone.

Stanko says, "Maybe we can give her Clonipine during the day for maintenance in a lower dosage."

"What do we do with Doug?" they say. "How do we keep him safe from Meggan?"

Stanko shakes his head. He opens his mouth, but the words simply do not surface.

There is nothing to say. He is a doctor, a human being from whom some sort of magic had been expected, whose bag of tricks, filled with medicine and logic, has been emptied. I wondered if Ken Stanko understood the extent of the Scanlons' disappointment, their feelings of letdown and betrayal. In fact, I led the discussion in that direction when he and I met privately the following week.

"It's entirely possible that without medication, things could be worse for Meggan," Stanko told me. If not for lithium and Tegratol, life might be a disaster. "It is also possible that the regimen requires additional adjustments . . . higher levels, for example, or a different or additional substance."

Establishing a regimen of medication for a psychiatric patient while in the hospital is never a "clean" experiment. By "clean" he is referring to the process of changing only one variable at a time, which is the usual objective. "You never change two medicines simultaneously, for example, because if something happens, good or bad, you are never sure which medication caused the change." Two variables were actually changed simultaneously at Western Psych during Meggan's most recent admission: the medication *and* the atmosphere—the simple fact that she was immersed in a highly structured living situation. She improved, "but it may have been the lithium and Tegratol and then again it may have been the strict hospital structure forced upon her. We can't be sure."

Another possibility is that Meggan's disintegrating behavior may simply be following the natural course of the illness. " 'Bipolar' means that her moods swing from one pole to another—from manic to depressed. Moods can be intense and prevalent at times, and then there are times when the situation is calmer." Meggan might have become hypomanic directly prior to her hospital admission. In the hospital, she stabilized. Three months later, soon after discharge, another cycle might have occurred. It is possible that Meggan's improved behavior had absolutely nothing to do with either the medication or the structure at Western Psych. She might have self-stabilized, independent of all intervention.

"Tom and Elizabeth must appreciate the ramifications of bipolar disease. They were so counting on things being better, so counting on the meds and the hospital to make the difference. And now, it is not happening as they had hoped. That's why," he said, referring to the previous session, "I attempted to prepare them for the worst."

It had been a tough session, but it was his responsibility to confront them with the facts and the prognosis especially in light of Meggan's joyride, a possible precursor to continually disintegrating behavior in the weeks and months to come. "Frustration is always proportional to expectation. One of my teachers taught me that little pearl. When we expect something and don't get it, we feel frustrated. The key is to lower your expectations, while preserving some hope for the future. Meggan is not over the edge yet."

He discouraged their thoughts about sending her away from home because they "were looking for the one and only answer. A place where their problems will be solved *for* them. There may be such a place, but I don't know where it is. We might hit it by accident, if we keep trying, and if we have unlimited funds, but there is no ideal destination. Meggan actually has a good chance to stabilize at home, if we can keep the situation from exploding." A number of long-range comparative studies confirm Stanko's assertion. R. M. Friedman and A. Duchnowski of the Florida State Mental Health Institute examined characteristics of mentally ill children placed in hospitals or residential care as contrasted to those treated while living at home, discovering that in the end there was little difference between the emotional well-being of the two groups.

One other crucial aspect was Meggan's absolute unwillingness to leave home under any circumstances. "Are the Scanlons prepared to throw their child out of the house?" Stanko wondered aloud. "I think not," he stated, answering his own question. Yes, it was possible to remove her, but could she be forced to behave, to study regularly, and to comply with medications? "I've heard adolescents say, 'If you send me to a boarding school, I'll run away. I'll get myself thrown out.'"

Nor was a group home a likely place for Meggan. Group homes and RTCs are usually equipped to stabilize kids *after* but not in lieu of the hospital experience. This was Dr. Boris's challenge in attempting to move Terri out of Mayview and Western Psych and into a group home, which is usually not prepared for patients with such an unpredictable and dangerous prognosis. And even if a group home or residential treatment center would accept Meggan, how could her parents afford to pay?

"The only other option for Tom and Elizabeth is the termination of parental rights, transferring the responsibility for her care, comfort, and future over to the state. That's a very hard thing to do—and undo. You are giving up your child forever. There's a good chance, even if you were to change your mind at a later date and want to reverse the ruling, that the Scanlons could never get Meggan back."

THE IDEA—the entire concept—of parents having to relinquish custody of their mentally ill or learning-disabled children in order to qualify them for the medical care and education that they need seems preposterous. This is a nugget of surrealistic humor snatched directly from the pages of Joseph Heller's novel *Catch-22*: ridiculous, outrageous, hilarious, farcical, but regrettably and tragically true. There are no statistics revealing how many parents have voluntarily relinquished custody of their children because they could not afford to care for them, but it is a regular occurrence across the nation.

In a seven-part award-winning series of investigative articles, entitled "A Child Apart: Troubled Youth, Troubled System," Frank Ritter, a reporter for the (Nashville) *Tennessean*, introduced his readers to Linda Steen. In the summer of 1988, Steen, thirty-eight, employment manager for the *Memphis Commercial Appeal* and a divorced mother of three facing bankruptcy because of the money expended for the unsuccessful treatment and hospitalization of her daughter, Marney, fourteen, "stood before a judge in Shelby County Juvenile Court and . . . asked the state to take over the mothering of her firstborn."

"Financially, I had no other choice. To get Marney the help she needed, I had to do what hurt the most—I had to give up custody of her."

The judge ordered an investigation of her family that was "humiliating and upsetting" and eventually denied her request, concluding that she was too good a parent to deserve help. "It was ironic . . . if I had been a negligent or abusive parent, they would have been quick to take her. I was asking, 'Why can't I, as a good parent, get the help I need? Why do I have to be a bad parent to get help?' " Ultimately, many months of battle and heartache later, Ms. Steen was able to relinquish custody of Marney. It was difficult enough having to commit such an act under public scrutiny, but to have to fight tooth and nail to receive permission to do so was ludicrous. Ms. Steen's request may have been granted, but that didn't mean she had won her battle or was in any way victorious.

"I didn't stop being her mother and I still 'mother' her to the extent that I can, but I had to give up the primary responsibility for parenting. I had to say, 'I am abandoning my child to get her the treatment she needs.' It was the most humiliating, frustrating, upsetting experience I have ever been through."

It would be nice to say that Ms. Steen's and Marney's sacrifices have been fruitful, but Marney has been transferred six times in a two-year period from juvenile detention to group homes to psychiatric wards in hospitals—with no apparent improvement in her condition. In essence, the state became Marney's keeper, just as the state or the county took Daniel away from his mother. But caring for these damaged kids and helping them get better so that they might one day reunite with their parents may well be an unobtainable goal in the near future without a reordering of health-care priorities in this country. It is also fair to say that such a reordering will not come to pass without a basic change in attitude toward mentally ill people. Would society tolerate a similar injustice, a relinquishment of parental custody, if Marney and Meggan had required kidney dialysis or heart surgery?

Although the Scanlons had their minds made up, Dr. Stanko wanted to shield them (and himself?) from the inevitable heartache and despair. "In my practice I've never had a situation where a family actually had to go to the state and say, 'We're going to terminate our parental rights. We can't take care of our kid, so we are going to let you do it.' " In his efforts to turn the parents away from relinquishment, he was attempting to respond to the needs of all three Scanlons rather than Meggan, Tom, or Elizabeth individually. "I can't imagine doing something for a patient that's not going to be helpful for the family as a whole. We're all in this together. We all have the same goal. We're on the same team. Everyone wants Meggan to feel better."

But Elizabeth Scanlon did not feel as if she were a part of Kenneth Stanko's team, as demonstrated at a meeting of Give Families a Break (GFAB), a support organization for parents with mentally ill children. GFAB has 450 families on its mailing list, but the organization's director, Lynn Alms, thinks there may be 35,000 people within a fifty-mile radius who would have some interest in being involved "if we could ever find them." She blames lack of membership on "the public stigma that goes along with psychiatric disorders. Schools and hospitals won't give out names and/or addresses because it constitutes a breach of confidentiality. Professionals—doctors, social workers, teachers—perpetuate the stigma of mental illness in this way."

As the meeting in late January begins, Elizabeth Scanlon introduces herself to the group, although some parents already know her, and says matter-of-factly that she has just devised the perfect way to win the war in the Persian Gulf that, at this point, has recently been initiated. "I am sending my daughter, Meggan, special delivery, to Saddam Hussein." Elizabeth's ability to joke in the face of her own despair continues to keep her going.

Briefing the rest of the families gathered here—perhaps twelve or fourteen people—Elizabeth says that Meggan has been home from Western Psych for a month "and we are beginning to feel really afraid."

Elizabeth says that the teachers at Winchester Thurston are so accommodating that she and her husband are beginning to question their judgment. "We're desperate to find a better place for her—a more therapeutic atmosphere, but our psychiatrist doesn't support us in our desire, so we are looking into it on our own. I admit we are not having much luck, however."

Pat, whose eight-year-old boy has a seizure disorder and is autistic as well, comments that her child has made a lot of progress over the past two years, but is now losing ground. He's getting too big and strong to handle, and he is becoming very aggressive.

Sally has a four-year-old autistic child. She, too, is beginning to recognize the possibility of aggression taking place in her child as time passes.

"Does he abuse your other children?" Pat asks.

"Not yet, but you can see it mounting," says Sally.

"Joey is pretty calm," says Donna, whose son is also autistic. "The only torment he goes through is in his own head."

In "A Child Apart," Frank Ritter has written about another Joey, who is ten years old, with a similar diagnosis, and the possible "scenarios for disaster" facing his thirty-seven-year-old single mother, Alice:

One scenario is that Alice will finally break under the crushing weight of unbelievable pressure. Her daily life, from the time she gets up in the morning to the time she goes to bed at night, is spent dealing with Joey, fighting to get him dressed in the morning, struggling to get him into the car that will drive him to school; coping with the behaviors that are at best inappropriate, at worst violent.

She can't even let him be alone in the home for any extended period of time. As with a three-year-old, she must constantly monitor his activities to keep him from, say, sticking his finger in an electrical outlet, running water in a sink until it overflows, or tearing a cover off an air conditioner.

Another scenario is that Joey, as he grows and matures, will become so strong and unruly that Alice will not be able to control him. Already, she worries whether he will hurt himself or someone else. She worries especially about his talk of suicide or bizarre fantasies. A third scenario for disaster—from Alice's standpoint—is that she might have to give up custody to get him into a program that would accommodate his needs.

If such a program exists.

John and Mary Ellen, veteran members of GFAB, have a nine-year-old boy, Jeff, who is autistic and suffers from a mood disorder. John is very upset, feels like his family is falling apart under the weight of Jeff's continuous demands. "This morning Jeff picked up a used prophylactic he found in a vacant lot, rubbed it all over his face, and then inserted it into his mouth."

John fears for his son's future. "What about when he's nineteen or even when he's twelve, when he cannot go to his school because that's the age limit, the extent of their facilities? There are articles in the paper about increased demands in child care for underprivileged families, but those articles are irrelevant to us because for autistic kids there is no child care at all!"

As the discussion travels around the circle of chairs and Styrofoam coffee cups, Elizabeth Scanlon says: "In every part of my life, I have always been a success, but I can't express to you how much of a failure I feel I am today. Meggan can cut into me with surgical precision, knowing instinctively the parts that will hurt the most."

Donna points out that Elizabeth's problems are more serious than the problems of most of the other parents gathered around the circle. "If you sit with my boy he will ask you the same question one hundred and fifty times, and sooner or later even the densest of people will understand that there is something significantly wrong with him. But nobody knows except you exactly what goes on in your house with Meggan."

"She looks perfectly normal," says Elizabeth. She selects a picture from a photo album and holds it up to show the group. "This is Meggan. She is incredibly charming when she wants to be."

Elizabeth continues to talk, exercising her unquenchable obsession to repeat her story time and again. As she talks, spewing forth each painful detail, she begins to cry, deep, silent sobs of frustration. "Basically my daughter is torturing us all the time." Elizabeth is wearing a blue cardigan sweater, the buttons of which she fingers nervously. "I am suicidal," she says. "That's all there is to it."

Donna asks if Meggan can get into Devereaux, a school for manic-depressive kids located in Philadelphia. This is one of the schools Stanko called "therapeutic boarding schools," but Meggan is actually doing well enough educationally at Winchester Thurston to eliminate such an expensive alternative. The school district and/or the state must be convinced that an education cannot be achieved in any other way in order to agree to pick up the tab. There are other group homes with schools, but "Meggan fools everyone into thinking that she's not the problem. Her parents are the problem," Elizabeth says.

Lynn Alms stresses that group homes are more aptly designed for kids in trouble—kids who have been neglected and abused, but not mentally ill. True, these kids might also have psychiatric problems, but the orientation is not congruent with treatment. There are host-homes programs—foster care for mentally disturbed children in people's houses. Ironically, foster families receive free psychiatric counseling for their kids, two weeks' respite care, access to recreational facilities, and constant caseworker support, along with a monthly stipend. Biological families of these same children would not receive any of these benefits.

"This is a slap in the face to the biological parents," says Pat. "If I got all of that help, I could live that way with my son for the rest of my life. We could manage." The system pulls families apart.

"I spent the weekend in my room," says Elizabeth Scanlon. "My husband brought me my meals on a tray. I have nothing to live for. I'm being controlled by this evilness inside and outside. I have been suicidal before, and I can tell you that I can't go on much longer. I'm filled with anger. I am a prisoner in my own home."

Someone asks about the help she is receiving from their psychiatrist.

"Dr. Stanko doesn't see it our way," says Elizabeth.

"That's because he's focusing on Meggan," says Nancy, "not you. You need someone to help you."

"Dr. Stanko says that nothing can be changed. That we cannot expect miracles, that Western Psych and the drugs have done everything they can. We have to live with her for the next five years and attempt to weather the storm with a minimal amount of conflict."

"What's he say you should do?" Pat asks, stomping her foot. Suddenly everyone is angry, screaming and yelling advice and criticizing Stanko.

"He said something about renting an apartment for her when she is seventeen," Elizabeth replies. This elicits even more anger from the group.

"You need to go to someone else if you expect to be alive for the next support group meeting."

"This may sound nitpicky," says John, "but it's important to remember that you actually don't hate your child. You hate your child's illness."

"And you hate your psychiatrist," Pat says. "Let him take care of Meggan himself for an afternoon, if he thinks that the situation is so easy to handle."

"But maybe it *is* us. Maybe we're not telling him right," says Elizabeth Scanlon. "Maybe we're at fault."

"We've all gone to twelve different doctors. Look around until you find someone who will help you and give you the support you need," John says.

"I'm too tired. I can't do this anymore. I've run out of doctors. I've run out of energy," says Elizabeth. "We've only been going to him for a month. Besides, there's no place to send her. Dr. Stanko was very highly recommended. What are we going to do?"

"As bad as it is," says Lynn, "this situation isn't as bad as it gets. Objectively speaking, you guys look pretty good compared to the desperate cases I've seen."

Donna gets up. She has to go home to Joey. She says to Elizabeth Scanlon, "I pray for you."

"Throw her out of the house," someone says.

"I don't want to throw her away," says Elizabeth Scanlon. "I want her to be happy and in a safe environment."

"But you have to *act* as if you do want to throw her away in order to get any attention at all, in this day and age. You should have refused to take her home from Western Psych in the first place," John says.

"I asked them if there was any option, if I could keep her there or send her anywhere else, and they said, 'No, this is the last stop.' I had to take her home."

"You could have refused." Another GFAB member whose daughter was also a manic actually refused to accept her child back. She finally received help and paid admission to Devereaux. "We're talking 'hard-ball' here," says John.

"The idea is, the way to fool the social workers is to look like you don't have any resources whatsoever. You are bone-dry," says Lynn.

"We don't really have any money left," says Elizabeth Scanlon.

"I mean emotional resources," Lynn says. "You have to be on the verge of destruction. The worst-case scenario."

"So where do you think I am?" Elizabeth asks.

"It's not where you really are, it's how the system perceives you that is most important."

Elizabeth is silent now. Her eyes are red and tears are streaming down her face. She has admitted her suicidal tendencies. She has told her story for God knows how many times to God knows how many people, and she seems to have been stopped in her tracks one more time without any reasonable option. People are supportive, but, like Stanko, they cannot make magic for her.

The discussion winds down. It is time to go home, to face the music of reality. They talk about IQs and how initially parents can be optimistic if their child's IQ is above the norm—it offers some hope. As time passes and the schools begin to fail them, IQs disintegrate, dropping 20 or 30 points in a few years. Jeff's IQ has fallen from 108 to a little above 80. In fact, if it falls a little more, Jeff can actually be considered mentally retarded and thereby receive all the services he cannot receive if he is a few points smarter, which is what a caseworker told Mary Ellen, John's wife, over the phone a couple of days ago. Mary Ellen replied, "I can't wait for my child to get stupider."

"Well," the caseworker replied, not recognizing the sarcasm, "that would certainly help."

Pat says, "If I had my choice I would take a Down's syndrome child any day over one with mental illness. Those kids are sweet. You can have a conversation with them. They may learn more slowly, but they want to learn and they want to please you, and they have a sense of what others feel. I swear to God, if I had it to do over again, I would choose, if I could make such a selection, a Down's syndrome child over a child suffering with a mental illness anytime."

MEGGAN'S DESCRIPTION of her driving adventure, as related to Dr. Stanko, sounds almost mystical.

"I was excited and extremely nervous. What if my parents came home when I was out? There was tension and suspense in the air. I went downstairs to the garage, and my heart was racing so fast, it was incredible. I took a couple of deep breaths. I knew I could do this. I would never get caught.

"I felt wonderful as I pulled out of the driveway and onto the street. Completely confident. I knew how to shift gears because I had studied my dad as he drove me to school. I knew when to shift because I had memorized the houses we passed as my dad shifted. I had even memorized the noise of the shifter and the clutch—I knew exactly the way it was supposed to sound when it was done right.

"Driving gave me an amazing feeling of happiness, although at the end I got scared because I realized I could have crashed and died."

She admitted that taking the car "was a stupid thing," but immediately justified her actions by pointing out that she knew exactly what she was doing. "Besides, it wasn't my fault. I needed help."

"As I understand it, you were home alone and watching television, and suddenly you were overcome with an urge to drive the car. You need help and support in controlling your impulses? Is that what you're saying?" Stanko asks.

"That's exactly what I told my dad," Meggan replies. "He should not have left the keys in the car."

"The keys were too tempting?"

"The keys were *very* tempting."

"You must always be aware of your goals, Meggan. As good as the driving made you feel for that moment, it set you back in terms of your goals, which are to get a driver's license when you turn sixteen and to be able to remain at Winchester Thurston." Stanko has frequently focused upon the goals he and Meggan have established during their discussions—a way of helping Meggan maintain a straight and narrow path.

When Tom, who has been waiting in the anteroom outside, is invited in, he announces that Elizabeth has decided to sever all communication with Meggan, including family therapy. He has been put in complete charge and has set severe limits. Meggan cannot go anywhere without money in her pocket. She must be home by six o'clock, no matter what. As Tom recites the new rules, he, as usual, becomes increasingly agitated, relating a series of complaints about Meggan.

Meggan turns to glare at her father. "Calm down," she says with a critical and overbearing parental tone.

"Meggan, he wasn't getting upset, he was just talking," Stanko tells her. Since the driving incident, Stanko seems to be hardening his opinion of and position toward Meggan.

Stanko and Tom begin to discuss Elizabeth's absence when Meggan suddenly interrupts. "Can't even take care of her own daughter," she says. "My mother doesn't care about me." Then she turns to Stanko. "My mother did this before. She left." Meggan is referring to a desperate time when Elizabeth left home and moved in with a girlfriend of hers.

Tom says to Meggan, "She is not leaving this time. She is trying to stay with us, but she needs some privacy and space."

"She won't even talk to her own daughter. Every time we get in the car, she starts to holler."

At the end of this session, and with Meggan's approval, Stanko announces that he will no longer separate the family—or in this case, Tom—during therapy. This action is in response to a conversation with Elizabeth's therapist, who, with Elizabeth's permission, had contacted him and informed him of her dissatisfaction with the way in which the therapy had been progressing. Stanko had telephoned Elizabeth and talked with her. They both agreed that she had become too distraught to continue to participate in family therapy. Stanko also learned that Elizabeth and Tom resented the fact that they had been banished from part of each session. Isolating the Scanlons had led to the misconception that he identified much more strongly with Meggan than he did with her mom and dad.

14

ELIZABETH SCANLON'S PERSONALITY initially overpowers her husband's quiet strength. I did not recognize nor appreciate the key role that Tom played as father, husband, and peacekeeper until our first in-depth private conversation, when Tom explained their dashed hopes and dreams.

"When we went to Western Psych, I was convinced there would be a break in the action. With medication, Meggan would become a sponge able to learn from her mistakes and move us beyond this state of constant war. But it's not happening. If anything, we're much more desperate than before. I can hardly believe what's in my mind—I'm literally ashamed for considering turning my back on my own child and walking away. Yet how can I turn my back on Elizabeth and Doug?

"Of all the people so far, Dr. Stanko seems to be the deafest. Maybe it's his style, and maybe he is attempting to be painfully honest, but Meggan comes home every night and beats us up verbally. Stanko advises us to avoid her attacks. It's like trying to avoid the air that's around you. What's worse, in the process of avoiding controversy, we have angered Meggan even further. Meggan told me, 'I'm going in Mom's room and I'm going to make her talk. I'm going to make her love me—no matter what.'

"Elizabeth is as close to shell shock as I've ever seen anybody and neither Stanko nor Meggan understands or cares. Meggan went skiing for the weekend. It was probably the best weekend we've had since she went to North Country School. Elizabeth, Doug, and I were giddy like little kids at Christmas the moment she left. Thursday night we all went out to dinner; we just sat there and talked and held hands and hugged and said how wonderful it was to have peace and quiet. We went out with a couple on Friday night for dinner, and Doug was just thrilled to stay home and have some quiet time. Saturday night he went skating with his girlfriend. We went to dinner and a movie. All the things that friends who have kids but who don't have a Meggan are doing. Nothing wild or crazy, just simple things.

"But when Meggan came home Sunday night and found out that we had bought clothes for Doug, she hit the roof. 'If you've got money for Doug, then you've got money to buy for me. I need a new pair of shoes'—a long list of demands. Elizabeth broke her silence, informing Meggan that if she could not behave herself, she would not be permitted to live in their house, to which Meggan replied: 'I'll drive you out of the house long before I leave. You'll have to call the police and forcibly remove me.'"

"You sit there and you stare, and you say, 'This is not good. This is not right. This is not the way people are supposed to live.'" He closes his eyes and then opens them again, looking around the room. "But then you realize, that's exactly how we have to live.

"Elizabeth refuses to go back and see Stanko. She has lost faith in him. I think in her heart of hearts she probably figures he's right. Maybe this is as good as it is going to get in the foreseeable future. But Stanko has given up—that's what we both feel. It must be comparable to how a cancer patient feels when a doctor says there's no hope. People want something to hang on to. According to Stanko, there's nothing left.

"I know I'm being unfair to Dr. Stanko. We are only paying him for an hour a week—and he's certainly giving us an hour of his undivided attention. I guess what it boils down to is that Meggan really needs daily therapy like she was getting at Western Psych. I try to help, but I'm not sure I know the right things to say. I don't know if anybody knows the right things to say to Meggan—or if there are right things to say.

"Meanwhile, I go home, and I'm scared to open the door. Like tonight. The kids are home. I hate to even think about what's happening. Stanko says that I should be prepared for the worst, go home assuming that they have thrown scalding water on each other, and beaten each other to a bloody pulp, so I'm not surprised when I finally find out the truth. But that's a crazy way to live. Meggan said to me last night, 'You're mad at me for being this way. I don't feel like I can be any different.'

"But I point out to her that Dr. Stanko believes that on a normal day-to-day basis the oppositional behavior is more her choice than a consequence of the disease. If she stabilizes in school, why is she at her worst with her mother, father, and brother? She says, 'I need to be able to vent my feelings and my anger somewhere, so when I get home, I feel like it is okay to explode.' "

Tom Scanlon smiles and shudders, as if he has had a sudden frightening notion. "Someone the other day told me about his manic-depressive sister. His parents get calls in the middle of the night about her from police departments and hospitals all over the country. Elizabeth and I know that this is probably where we're headed unless something dramatic changes—soon. Meggan may leave the house at eighteen, but she will be just as abrasive and irritating with employers as with us. She'll hold it together for a while—until the employer asks her to work overtime. Then she'll let fly with her world-famous tirade and will be out of a job.

"We're going to have to decide whether we're going to turn our backs on her or bail her out when she's in trouble. When she marries somebody and abuses them the way she's abused us, it's possible she's going to be a battered wife. When the story unfolds, we'll have to sit there and say, 'Yeah, I felt like doing exactly what he did many times myself.' How can I look at her husband or boyfriend and be angry because they hit my baby, when I will know how furious he felt inside and how she pushed him and taunted him?

"Dr. Cohen used to say that I'm allergic to conflict, so I manage to avoid dealing with an awful lot. Maybe this makes me a real shallow person, but the funny thing is, even though I just spent the last two hours spilling my guts about how miserable my life is, I could probably go out right now, meet a friend, and take in a baseball game—and not think about Meggan for a moment. I'm not sure how I do that, but I am lucky to be that way. My ability to tuck Meggan back into the far recesses of my mind is the primary reason I've been able to successfully maintain my sanity. Otherwise, I'd be blown-out and dead."

AT THE BEGINNING of February, one of those brief and beautiful honeymoon periods occurs when all of Elizabeth's, Tom's, and Meggan's efforts, along with the medications and the talk treatment, seem to jell. That therapeutic elixir called "hope" is in the air.

Today, Tom Scanlon is smiling, and he sinks into Stanko's easy chair with an aura of confidence, as if he expects to enjoy the next fifty minutes. "This has been a good week. No major flare-ups." He looks at Meggan. "You are getting yourself out of bed on time. You only stayed up late one night." Then he looks back at Stanko. "Even then, she did not get into our space."

"Why do you think it was such a good week?" Stanko asks.

Tom smiles at Meggan. "I wonder if it has something to do with what we have been explaining to you recently," says Tom. "That if your flare-ups continue, you might not be living with us anymore?"

Meggan does not reply directly, but instead begins to recite the list of goals she and Dr. Stanko have developed over the weeks, including "driving at sixteen, not leaving home, passing all of my courses at school." Meggan's poor performance in school—the one arena in which she has in the past been effective—continues to be worrisome. Tom has been in regular contact with Meggan's teachers, informed of her progress on a weekly basis. Quite gratuitously, the school has decided that because of her hospitalization whatever grades Meggan earns for the second semester will count for the entire school year.

But her teachers have reported that Meggan seems increasingly confused, not passing tests or handing in homework assignments—facts to which she is completely oblivious. Meggan seems to believe that her responsibilities at school are being fulfilled, that her work is up-to-date and competent. Meggan has flatly denied her documented grades, *D*s and *F*s. When Tom and Dr. Stanko quizzed her, Meggan could not remember her class schedule or the names of some of her teachers, or connect teachers with a subject. The principal reported that she had discovered Meggan sitting in her office one morning. "I have to telephone my father about a doctor's appointment," she said. Meggan was sent to class and told to contact her father at lunch, a more appropriate time for telephoning.

"Why are you late?" the teacher had asked when Meggan arrived.

"Because," she replied, "I missed my bus."

Meggan spent most of the previous weekend with her friend Laura, ostensibly doing homework. But when she returned home Sunday evening she suddenly realized that she had a Monday-morning test and needed Laura's notes to prepare. Meggan phoned Laura, who said that she would need her notes before school because that was when she planned to study. Meggan's solution to this dilemma was to take a 5:00 A.M. bus to Laura's house, thus using Laura's notes before her friend got out of bed.

Tom and Elizabeth went along with Meggan's "poor judgment" because it was consistent with Stanko's treatment plan: to go to bed at 10:00 P.M., to be at school on time, to take her medications, to turn in her assignments. Those were the challenges and guidelines. How she managed them was her business, as long as her methods were not dangerous and destructive.

Meanwhile, Tom was beginning to question the appropriateness of Winchester, where "Meggan is like a square peg in a round hole." Both Stanko and Debbie Rubin had privately questioned the choice of Winchester from the beginning. "It was," Debbie Rubin had said, "a reflection of where the Scanlons had hoped Meggan could go to school, not founded in any semblance of reality."

But Tom does not want to give up on Winchester—not yet— especially considering the positive change in Meggan over the past week. Stanko had suggested that they stop waking Meggan in the morning because getting her out of bed precipitated arguments. Meggan had to learn how to be responsible for her own schedule. This morning she slept in. Realizing that she was very late, she tried to persuade her father to drive her to school. Tom refused. Normally Meggan would have attempted to browbeat him until he capitulated. "But today, she respected what I said, somehow got it together, and actually caught the bus. This for Meggan is quite an accomplishment."

Stanko is very excited hearing this story. He leans forward, smiling and cocking a finger: "How did you do it, Meggan? How did you get it together? Did you think of all of your goals? Did you think to yourself, 'I want to drive when I am sixteen, and this is a golden opportunity to demonstrate to my father how responsible I am'?"

"That's exactly what I thought," Meggan says.

At the end of the session, Stanko skillfully summarizes the good things that have happened during that week and the problems that remain. Because of the absence of a confrontational and crisis atmosphere, for the first time the session ends on time.

ON FEBRUARY 20 the Scanlon roller coaster hits bottom. Tom stomps into Stanko's office, angry and red-faced. "Okay, it's rug-cutting time. We're down to it now. We have to make decisions here, and we have to make them quick. The gun is going off. My head is exploding." He points across the room at Meggan. "She got up this morning and announced that she wasn't going to go to school anymore. She quit! This is too much! I'm not equipped to deal with someone who is going to quit. I don't have any money anymore, and my daughter has just quit school. This is insane.

"I sat down at the dinner table last night and asked Doug how he was doing. I haven't had the chance to say a word to Doug because I've been so embroiled in Meggan's problems. But at that moment, Meggan got jealous and angry, picked up her plate, and said, 'I don't want to sit and listen to this talk about his fucking A grades.'

"Well, I've had it," says Tom. "That's all I really have to say. I'm sitting here now and asking you for help. At this point I'm in a panic, Doctor. I was in tears this morning because my kid tells me that she is quitting school. I don't know what to do."

Stanko is calm and rational, replying in an even, careful tone. But it is clear that his sympathies have turned, that he is beginning to value and acknowledge the Elizabeth-and-Tom side of the Scanlon equation. "Meggan needs structure and well-defined goals."

"But haven't you told us to back off and give her space? What do you say about that contradiction?" Before Stanko can answer, Tom continues, less harshly: "What I'm saying is that I don't have the tools to take care of Meggan anymore. She needs a keeper—not a parent." He leans back in his chair, as if he is finished speaking, but then, thinking of another topic, he leans forward. "And what in the hell are we going to do this summer? Elizabeth can't quit her job. We need the money. But if Meggan is home and her brother is home, then World War III will occur in our living room. Last summer, Meggan was left alone and she had sexual experiences with people she hardly knew."

Stanko remains respectfully attentive. "It may be that Meggan's quitting school reflects her own realization that she can't make it there. If that's what she is realizing, then we have to face it. You mentioned the same possibility in this room just last week."

"That's right," says Tom. "But I am not going to let her sit at home until next September."

Suddenly, Meggan interrupts angrily, saying that she knows that Elizabeth is secretly trying to send her away to school. "I just want to make it clear that I am not for any reason leaving the house."

"So that's your ultimatum?" Tom says.

Up to this point and in fact through most of their sessions, Stanko has been very withdrawn, generally reluctant to assert himself and disrupt the dynamics between father and daughter. But clearly, the extent of conflict and frustration has reached a breaking point.

"Meggan is not in a position to give ultimatums," he says suddenly, surprisingly loudly. He then turns to Meggan. "Whether you stay at home until you are nineteen, or whatever age, is not your decision, it's your parents'."

"I know," she says. "I am supposed to achieve my goal to stay at home by working hard."

"That's what this is all about," Stanko exclaims, spreading his arms. "Your goals are not unrealistic. These are reasonable plans. You have to give it your best shot. You want to stay home? You have to be cooperative and compliant. Otherwise, you may well suffer the consequences."

There is a long silence now. I'm not sure how much of an impact Stanko has made, but Meggan seems to understand that even though she does not want to leave home, if she continues to misbehave she might very well have to. The session ends quietly. Meggan doesn't seem to know how to proceed.

A WEEK LATER, Stanko immediately announces that there are two important items on the agenda. "The first relates to the medication you have been taking, Meggan. Have you felt any changes in your behavior since I decreased your lithium?" Noticing that Meggan's lithium blood levels had been higher, Stanko had decreased the amount of medication that had been prescribed since her hospital discharge. "Any change in your sleep patterns? How about your overall mood for the past week?"

"I can't remember," Meggan says. "But I can't concentrate. That I can tell you. I can't think things out. My mind wanders. I'm always doing something silly in my head."

"Concentration has been a problem for you for a while," Stanko notes, as he flips through her file. "It's hard to tell if medication is making that better or worse. Your mom and dad told me that you were considerably more irritable, hyper, and emotional over the past week."

"I don't remember," Meggan replies. "I actually don't know what they are talking about."

"That's another reason that your mood is so difficult to evaluate. Other people assess your behavior differently than how you see yourself."

Since entering the room, Meggan has been squirming in her chair, laughing, and making whimpering noises. "Is that bad?"

"Not bad, but it's hard to know what to do about the problem."

"Maybe I am a split personality." She laughs, sits up, and gazes out the window.

"The second thing on the agenda," Stanko says, then hesitates, shakes his head, and begins again. "It would be much simpler, Meggan, if the medication was actually the cause of our problems. We would find the correct number and combination of pills and the situation would be hunky-dory. But your parents and I are beginning to realize that the problem is more complicated. This screaming and haranguing that you have been doing . . . Your parents think . . ." Stanko hesitates again.

Meggan suddenly sits up, and turns angrily away from the window to glare at her father. "I won't leave the house," she announces. "Don't even think of considering it."

Stanko does not seem to be deterred by his patient's strong objection. "Well, Meggan, as we discussed last week, that won't be your decision. Your parents have the responsibility to do something, if your behavior is not in the family's best interests—"

Once again, Meggan interrupts. "But what am I supposed to do about that? It is not my fault."

"Well, you are asking the right question," says Stanko. "I hear you. But it has nothing to do with fault. It is your first question that we have to think about. What can you do about your behavior? If you really want to live at home, what can you do to help achieve that goal? Because, Meggan, you need to know that your goal of staying at home is in serious jeopardy."

Now Meggan slumps down in her chair, turns back toward the window, and stares, lonely and vacant. It is a clear, cloudless day. The sun streaming through the window paints a broad yellow band on Stanko's desk.

"You're awful quiet, Meg. You have to talk," Tom says.

"What's there to say? I am trying my hardest. You guys aren't helping me a bit. What have you ever done to help me, except send me to a bunch of stupid psychiatrists all my life?"

Stanko explains the distinction between the help they have given, such as therapy and private schools, and the fact that it hasn't worked. "You can't say your parents haven't tried, it's just not been as successful as they had hoped."

Meggan contends that her parents are expecting too much. Do they want her to do well at school or at home? "I can't concentrate on both." She points at her father. "If he wants me to get good grades, I can't be a good daughter. And if he wants me to be a great daughter, I can't get good grades."

"Great choice!" Tom says.

Stanko turns toward Tom, shrugs, and spreads his arms, as if to say that Meggan is making sense, that this might just be the exact choice Tom and Elizabeth will be forced to make. Perhaps Meggan is at her best. By this time, Meggan has slumped so low in her chair that her back and head are flat on the seat, and she is squirming around and whining, her hands covering her face.

"Well, if you have a choice between passing the ninth grade or living at home, what would you choose?" Stanko asks.

"Stay at home." She adds that she also doesn't want to leave Winchester Thurston—"WT," she calls it—where all her friends are. Not now or next semester, either.

Stanko is sympathetic. "It must be difficult to go from school to school, make new friends, and then lose those friends again. But we can't discuss where you're going to school next year just yet, because if things don't get better at home, your very first goal, which is staying at home, won't be possible."

"I am not leaving home," Meggan says.

"I don't know why you are saying that, Meggan," says Tom. "Don't you always tell me, 'I'm fine as long as I am not with any of you'? So now you have the chance to get out. Besides, I'm not certain that I believe that you really can't control your behavior. Sometimes I think you are oppositional on purpose."

Meggan looks surprised, and then smiles.

"Is that true? Are you sometimes oppositional on purpose?" Stanko asks.

Meggan shrugs. "Well, it works."

For a moment, Stanko pauses, chuckles, and nods. "But, Meggan, there's one problem. It works, but it is also inconsistent with living at home, which is your goal. You cannot keep annoying your parents if you want to stay at home. You need to think this out more clearly, Meggan. You need to think! Think! Think about your goals."

Now he leans forward and whispers loudly and dramatically, "Can't get a car if you're not at home. Can't get a driver's license if you're not at home. Can't go to Winchester if you're not at home. What's important for you to understand is that your parents' goal is the exact same goal as yours, which is for you to stay at home. If you do not stop irritating them, neither of you will achieve your goals."

"They want me out of the house," Meggan says.

Stanko replies, "I don't believe that, Meggan."

"No, Meggan. We don't want you out of the house," Tom says softly. "That's not what we want."

Meggan shakes her head, yawns, and turns back toward the window. "I am so tired. I am currently so tired. I have to go home to get some rest."

LATER, in compliance with the Scanlons' wishes, Kenneth Stanko contacted Children and Youth Services (CYS) to investigate the possibility of placing Meggan outside of the home. Contact with CYS is usually handled by a social worker attached to a facility, such as Debbie

Rubin at Western Psych. Stanko, who might talk with a CYS representative once every two or three years, dialed the main number and was connected with a supervisor whom he did not know, to whom he outlined the Scanlon family difficulties. The supervisor promised to look into the situation and call him back, but neither the supervisor nor Stanko could offer the Scanlons much hope of cooperation.

15

PERIODICALLY, I met with Ken Stanko for informational discussions so that I could understand his approach to family therapy and to the Scanlons' case specifically. In these discussions, Dr. Stanko was always candid and thorough. We discussed the wisdom of initially separating Meggan from her parents during the session, a decision of which I had been skeptical and which he had finally reversed. Didn't separation in therapy actually polarize the two factions rather than enhance togetherness and trust?

Trust was actually a reason for his action, Stanko explained, particularly important when the parents—not the child—had selected the doctor. Time alone with Meggan was essential to gain her confidence. Would Meggan tell him secrets she didn't want her parents to know? What if she became pregnant? Felt suicidal? Contemplated running away? It was important she believed that a confidential conversation with her doctor was possible.

Stanko understood that the Scanlons resented the separation, suspecting that he was only hearing Meggan's side of their dispute, which may have been true periodically. "But it is not necessary for a therapist to receive a blow-by-blow description of everything that happens." Such reportage would take forever—"and it is not going to change my treatment plan. I don't need to know all these details." Stanko routinely assumes "some distortion, some concealing" in the information provided by patients. "The instance about driving the car and hitting the garage? I heard Meggan's story, and I know that when compared to a video of that night, her version would be a bit different. That's okay. It's only a problem if there are serious lies and distortions—and it's hard not to know when the person you are talking to is pathological."

His decision to become a "buffer" between Meggan and her parents was "absolutely necessary. This was one way of helping redirect the 'war' between Tom and Elizabeth and Meggan *at me* and away from the family in order to decrease tension between them."

But how could an hour of therapy a week, plus phone calls for crisis situations, change people who had been at odds for fifteen years—especially considering Elizabeth's and Tom's states of mind?

"It probably can't, but I had to try," Stanko replied. Besides, he had hoped that Meggan's medication, when properly adjusted, might decrease her irritability and impulsiveness. While waiting for the medication to do its work, his "buffer" role would provide a temporary reprieve. "This same approach has worked for me many times."

"You expected many phone calls?"

He nodded. "I entered into the situation with my eyes open." The plan didn't work not because of Meggan, Tom, or Elizabeth individually, but because of their inability to overcome past behavioral patterns. Meggan needed to stabilize her moods, while Tom and Elizabeth had to detach themselves from Meggan's every action. With medication, Meggan's moods were perhaps "only a tiny bit unstable," but her parents, so sensitized to her unpredictable nature, often overreacted to potentially harmless situations, which in turn triggered instability from Meggan. Stanko drew a simple circular diagram, illustrating the Meggan-Tom-Elizabeth "vicious cycle" in which Meggan's moods and her parents' response fueled each other and stimulated an irreversible and escalating chain of destructive events.

"What specifically starts it? Is it Meggan, Tom, or Elizabeth who is responsible for initiating the trouble? Who cares?" said Stanko, throwing up his arms and shaking his head. "You can spend a lot of time trying to answer that question, but it doesn't matter. Somehow, the cycle is triggered and all three participants are doing battle, suddenly out of control. What is really important is how it can be interrupted. Because as soon as we break the cycle, either through the parents or the patient, the bad behavior and the escalating situation will stop."

Thus it was Kenneth Stanko's determination that by making himself a buffer between the warring factions he could interrupt the cycle, thereby de-escalating the situation. Perhaps peace talks—discussions leading toward understanding and compromise—might begin. But his efforts had not been successful; he could not interrupt the cycle, which had a life and a fuse of its own. Two healthy adults without fifteen years of emotional combat behind them might have been able to turn the corner successfully, but Tom and Elizabeth were too far gone. On the other hand, it is also possible that Meggan's biology would not allow her to cooperate and break the cycle. "There is an old saying: The patient says, 'I cannot'; others say, 'She will not.' The truth is that the patient 'cannot will.' "

ANOTHER ISSUE THAT Stanko and I examined was his personal feelings toward the Scanlon family, especially in light of the fact that the Scanlons harbored some resentment toward his approach to their case. Stanko explained the Freudian concept of "transference," in which the patient attributes to the therapist repressed feelings about others in his life. "Countertransference" represents therapists' feelings and thoughts toward their patients during the therapeutic experience. "You learn to expect countertransference and at the same time to not permit it to interfere. When I become aware of feelings of irritation toward my patient, I just say to myself, 'My job is to be here with this patient—no matter what horrors he or she may be relating to me concerning his or her own behavior.' " Sometimes Stanko will utilize the "Just Say No to Drugs" approach to eliminate his own errant thoughts. "It may not be successful as a social policy, but it can sometimes be helpful for individual patients and problems."

"Feelings can be so overpowering," Stanko told me one day. "Psychiatrists have lots of different feelings toward their patients: sadness, worry, anger, or sexual attraction—but we try to keep them separate from what we're doing professionally.

"In relation to the Scanlons, I may have felt, 'Oh my God, there's a meeting at Western Psych' [referring to a case discussion scheduled by Debbie Rubin which he has been asked to attend]. That's two hours out of my day, two hours I won't get paid. I don't *feel* like doing that. But I know it would be helpful and supportive, so that feeling doesn't determine my decision." He agreed to attend the meeting, but also decided to charge a consultation fee. "The fact that I was going to get some legitimate compensation helped assuage resentment."

I said that I understood the distinction between feelings and how he refused to allow them to affect his behavior or interfere with his treatment, but this didn't really explain how he actually felt about the Scanlons as people.

"There's a difference between getting feelings about a patient and getting feelings in a session *with* a patient," he said. As an example, he can be irritated because he scheduled a late appointment on a day when he would really rather go home to play with his kids. In this situation, his feelings may have nothing to do with the Scanlons, or whomever the patient happens to be. Stanko admitted that "there were times when I felt definite irritation toward the Scanlons, but when I examined my irritation it had to do with things like trekking into Western Psych and taking that chunk of time; I just do not enjoy going to meetings." But his irritation toward the Scanlons didn't stop there.

"There were times I felt irritated when the Scanlons would call me at home. They would call my answering service, which would ring me: 'Doctor, we have an emergency. Please call Elizabeth and Tom Scanlon right away.' Now, I am in the middle of playing with my kids—and I get irritated almost any time that happens, regardless of who the patient is.

"But there was a period when it happened a fair number of times. So I would feel irritated because it was interfering with my life." On the other hand, he admits that if he offers his patients his telephone availability, he must be on hand in crisis situations. But that knowledge and responsibility will not necessarily make him feel better when the crisis and the subsequent phone call it triggers occur.

One thing that does help him control his irritation in such a situation, that allows him to change immediately into a "work mindset," is the fact that he will be getting paid for his overtime efforts. He will bill a patient for time on the telephone, "although," he added sheepishly, "I didn't in the case of the Scanlons."

Typically, Stanko explained, he will keep track of his phone time, and when he has accumulated an hour's worth, he will say something like, "I am not telling you not to call me; I want to offer my help whenever you need me. But I will have to bill you as though it were a session." He doesn't have a stopwatch on his desk, and he is not as rigid as, say, lawyers, because there is another objective running through his mind: building a good relationship with his patients. If for any reason a strong foundation has not been established, he will often give extra time in his office or on the telephone without charging. "I was right at that point with the Scanlons when I would have told them it was time to pay."

This is one of the most perplexing problems of practice psychiatrists face, especially in such a personal and competitive field, in which a slip of the tongue or an unwise decision may cost a physician a client (patient) who might have spent a month, or a year, in therapy. "I sit there with the Scanlons and other patients and say to myself, 'Okay, we really went overtime today. Should I bring up the subject of billing?' " Many of his Scanlon sessions went ninety minutes or longer "but I made a conscious decision to not charge extra because it was too risky. I could have given the wrong impression. 'Gee, all he's thinking about is getting paid. He's watching the clock and he wants to get paid. He really isn't that interested in us.' That's what they might have thought—and it wasn't true.

"So I didn't bill the Scanlons for their telephone calls, even though I knew it would make me feel better, because I wanted to make sure that the relationship was stable enough so that when I finally asked for the money, they would understand and agree that I deserved it."

For her book *Psychoanalysis: The Impossible Profession*, Janet Malcolm conducted a series of interviews with an analyst she calls Aaron Green, experiencing similar financial conflicts. Green tells Malcolm of a dinner with friends, non-analysts, one evening in which someone jokingly began discussing psychiatrists' fees, a subject about which Green is extraordinarily sensitive. "I frankly want more money than I have," he tells Malcolm, "and I am envious of analysts who are rich, yet I can't bring myself to do what is necessary to increase my income, that is, beg for referrals. So I have unfilled hours, and I am bitter."

He then tells a story about a patient whom he saw daily, and who did not pay for eight months. Green continued therapy essentially as a symbol of trust, despite the hardship it caused and the festering resentment. "I consider it one of the most heroic things I have ever done as an analyst and it was tremendously successful." One day the patient appeared with a check for the entire amount, but now he has stopped paying again, a source of tension and worry. "So when they started making jokes about fees at the dinner party, I wasn't disposed to laugh, and I began very earnestly and seriously to explain to them how very important these things are." His friends continued to joke "and finally I committed the grossest social faux pas. I lashed out with the most boorish, pontificating, morally outraged tirade—embarrassing everyone there, and most of all me. There I was, an analyst—mature, reflective, well-analyzed (more or less)—acting just like a person. Worse."

For obvious reasons, psychiatrists are expected to demonstrate behavior and maturity above and beyond the norm, especially in situations in which most humans are typically vulnerable and fragile. Ken Stanko is finding it increasingly difficult to balance his responsibility as a professional and his need to earn a living and remain intertwined with his family. The comments of his wife, Anne Muscarella, might resemble a story that one of his patients could tell.

"When my husband comes home, it's seven o'clock, sometimes later, and he tries to give his kids time and attention—I often think he tries too hard to make up for the time he doesn't see them. He also tries to please me; he does the dishes when he can, and the laundry. But his telephone time begins officially at nine o'clock. That phone, I keep telling him, is one of the biggest strains on the marriage. We have to find a way of changing that situation. We need more together time, and the problem is, if we wait until eleven o'clock for time to talk, do you think he feels like talking? I know he wants to be alone.

"I am very hesitant to unload on him, like one of his patients—but I have a lot of frustrations, coping with the kids and the house, and everything during the day. What seems to be happening is that we have stretches in which there is a lot of distance between us that shouldn't really be there. When his practice was slower and he wasn't so busy, we had more time." Anne Muscarella also finds it difficult to argue with someone whose communication skills are so fine-tuned. "As a psychiatrist, he argues skillfully. He can express himself better than I can. His point will always sound more valid than my point, even when I am sure my point is just as valid—or he is wrong. And that is annoying and frustrating. Ken can also get very irritable; he is a high-strung Type A personality, especially when he is tired; he will bend with the strain—and snap. For a long time, I would take it personally, but I know he doesn't mean any harm. Anger is short-lived with him. I can't even think of a time when it has lasted more than an hour. So things don't go well for us all of the time; we have issues and problems like everyone else. But we have a foundation and a purpose. Our values and our commitments to religion and to family will keep us together no matter how much distance has been created."

GUESS WHAT?" says Meggan on March 6. "I'm going into the hospital on Friday." She begins naming all of the people—Dr. Boris, Debbie Rubin, and her nurse, Don Svidergol—whom she will be seeing at Western Psych.

"What about them?" Stanko asks. Clearly, he is taken aback, unaware that events have unfolded so quickly and without his consultation.

"They are my family."

Slumping down into her chair, Meggan observes in a scattered manner that she has always known deep in her heart that she would end up back in the hospital. "I dream about going back to the hospital all the time," she says. "Dreaming about how good it is to come out of the hospital with everyone liking me again. It's a wonderful feeling. I always knew it would happen."

Stanko says, "What do you hope will happen in the hospital?"

"I hope that they will put me on some medication so I can learn to concentrate and get through school. I hope they will teach me not to fight. You see," she says, "if I get better medications then I'll be able to drive better, and if I drive better then I won't have any accidents." Meggan is squirming in her chair, stretching toward the window, rambling and mumbling in a monotone.

"How can the medication help you?" Stanko interrupts.

"The medication will change my brain around. My brain has got to get organized. There's nothing I can do about it." She rambles on about her uncontrollable behavior. Her voice trails off.

"Do you know how long you'll be in the hospital?" asks Stanko.

"Two months."

"Then what?"

"Go back to school. See how it works out."

"Then it will be summer," says Stanko. "You won't be able to go back to school."

"I can get out of Western Psych in a month then. I will go back to school and see everybody."

"Are you scared, Meggan?"

"I'm not worried about it anymore. I have ninety people coming to visit me. Melissa is there already." She is referring to an old roommate at Western Psych.

"But what if the medication in the hospital can't solve your problems, like you want it to?"

"Then I will have to do it myself," she says.

"How will you do it?"

"I'll have to . . . if I can. I hope I can. I know I can. Unless there's something wrong with me. But there's nothing wrong with me. Unless . . ." There's a long silence. Suddenly she says, "I'm hungry. I need to eat."

Stanko is clearly dismayed, not nearly as animated as usual. His shoulders are hunched. Nobody seems to want to talk. The silence goes on for long seconds until Meggan starts to laugh.

"My stomach is growling." She laughs again.

Tom says, "This laissez-faire approach that you wanted us to take—backing off, letting Meggan make some of her own mistakes—is easier said in the calm of this office than done in real life."

"I appreciate that," says Stanko, "but it can work." He turns to Meggan. "I don't know how long they will let you stay in the hospital."

"I can stay as long as I want," says Meggan.

"Meggan, that's not your decision," says Stanko. "What will you do about it when they tell you to leave?"

"I'll go home."

"That might not be your decision either," he tells her.

Soon after, Meggan leaves the office to meet her mother in the parking lot.

"What will your role be from now on?" Tom says to Stanko.

"When she goes to the hospital, Dr. [Boris] Birmaher is her physician."

"But you're her doctor, and you should be part of the team."

"I'll be as much a part of the team as you want me to be," Stanko says.

Surprisingly, Tom seems very upset. Perhaps he has changed his mind, believing that Dr. Stanko was actually beginning to make progress with Meggan. Or maybe he has simply become attached to Stanko during all these weeks, realizing that Stanko had ended up identifying with the parental problems he and Elizabeth had been experiencing.

"You and Elizabeth should feel free to call me," Stanko says in a clear and steady voice.

"We will," Tom replies, as the two men stand and shake each other's hands in a stiff and formal manner. "I can't say that it's been a pleasure." He smiles. "But . . . thanks."

DANIEL

I SAW LESS and less of Daniel over the next year but we kept in touch by meeting periodically at the local Pizza Hut. He was changing.

One Saturday, he arrived with a hunting knife in a sheath on his belt—"for protection." He said he was making new friends, such as Big Tim, the devil-worshiper, and Jonesy, the skinhead Nazi. Daniel also had his own street name, "Pony Boy." He had hooked up with a gang he referred to as "the posse," but "its official name is the KKK." Daniel had never heard of the Ku Klux Klan and did not know what it stood for. They were his friends, he said.

I did not see Daniel again for a long time, but when we next got together at the Pizza Hut he had just come back from running away. He had met a girl who was being abused at home by her father, and he told her that he had a secret house where they could both live. The place was a figment of Daniel's imagination, an idea that had evolved recently; he had a home, a car, and a job. This was also part of his ever-increasing "rescue" fantasy, the idea that he, the daring do-gooder, could impact upon the lives of others while controlling his own.

Daniel and his girlfriend spent the night in the woods, necking and shivering in the freezing rain. The police found them the following morning, wet and dirty.

"That sounds like a pretty senseless adventure."

"Yeah." Daniel laughed. "So many of the things I do are dumb."

That day, Daniel wanted to talk about his sixteenth birthday, because he could then apply for work at McDonald's.

"Some people say that I won't amount to anything," he said, "but I will show them what I can do. Maybe I can't read and write, but I can work two or three jobs if I have to. I want a family and a car and my own house, and I'll do anything it takes to be like normal people. Don't you think that that's possible, if I try real hard?"

"Nobody tries as hard as you do, Dan," I told him.

"Then you think I can have a normal life?"

"You bet," I lied.

PART FIVE

Stuck in Time

16

AS DEBBIE RUBIN waited in her office for the Scanlons to arrive for their first family therapy session since Meggan's readmission, she pondered the complexity of the situation they must confront: Elizabeth and Tom seemed unable to accommodate their dreams for Meggan with reality. School was an ideal example of the dichotomy of their feelings. On the one hand, they insisted that they didn't care about Meggan's daily achievement; it would be okay if Meggan did not graduate from high school until she was twenty-five and worked the rest of her life at a hardware store. Yet instead of providing an unpressured educational atmosphere, they thrust her into the challenging and competitive academic world of Winchester Thurston. And to make matters worse, they became angry when Meggan admitted she could not cut it, even though she was telling them the truth. How many times had they voiced their frustration because their daughter would not be honest? The Scanlons had to learn to give a more uniform message to Meggan and to modify their expectations.

A similar situation had occurred in relation to Meggan and her ill-fated driving experience. Meggan had a history of impulsivity and opposition combined with an absolute lust to drive. Meggan was left alone in the house, tempted by car keys dangling in the ignition. Not that Tom and Elizabeth had baited Meggan, but they had not been realistic about Meggan's need for structure and control. The keys should not have been made so temptingly available.

"What quality of behavior is reasonable to expect from Meggan?" Debbie Rubin wondered aloud. "That she go to school every day? Probably. That she go to bed on time every night and treat her family with respect? Well, probably not." But how to convince Tom and Elizabeth to understand that "this may be as good as it gets"?

"The worst part of my job, the saddest and the hardest, is sitting with a parent and telling them that the kid is seriously emotionally disturbed and there is little to be done about it. It is right up there with telling somebody that their kid has cancer. Life isn't fair. You try to be a good parent and do everything right, but sometimes things just don't work out."

Dr. Boris, who joined the Scanlons that day for family therapy, began by questioning the validity of Meggan's bipolar diagnosis. After all, she had not responded to traditional lithium/Tegratol treatment. Years ago, Meggan had once been diagnosed with attention deficit hyperactivity disorder (ADHD), but because of her positive scholastic achievements, the diagnosis had been minimized. "Perhaps it has finally reached an uncontrollable state," Dr. Boris said.

The Scanlons, sitting in Debbie Rubin's office, seeking clarity concerning diagnosis and treatment, were then presented with a number of mixed messages. The first order of business was to wean Meggan from all medications and watch for the manic episode required to confirm a bipolar diagnosis. When Meggan was "clean," Ritalin, the traditional medication for hyperactivity, might be introduced. If Meggan's behavior then stabilized, perhaps she was actually not bipolar but hyperactive, thus showing Ritalin as an effective mode of treatment. Stabilized behavior might also indicate that Meggan was simply not experiencing a manic or hypomanic period, however—Meggan could be either bipolar or ADHD. On the other extreme, Ritalin has been known to trigger bipolar episodes.

"So what this all means," Elizabeth told Debbie Rubin after Dr. Boris departed, "is that we are playing mix and match with drugs and diagnosis all over again."

"So once again the doctors have cured Meggan Scanlon," Debbie

Rubin announced. "But of course, they've already cured her a hundred times before. What else is new?"

IN THE MOVIE *The Blues Brothers*, John Belushi and his cohort Dan Aykroyd, attempting to save a church school from extinction, believe they are on a mission from God, which is how William Pelham, who had just earned his Ph.D. in psychology at the University of Florida, describes his own orientation in the late 1970s. "I was on a mission from God to prove that psychiatric medication was bad for kids and that behavior modification was better."

Pelham was referring to the fact that Ritalin (the brand name for methylphenidate, a stimulant similar to Dexedrine) has long been used for kids suffering from ADHD. At that time, Peter Schrag and Diane Divoky had debunked hyperactivity in their controversial book, *The Myth of the Hyperactive Child*, while another widely discussed book, by Benjamin Feingold, *Why Your Child Is Hyperactive*, speculated that hyperactivity might be controlled by restricting food additives and sugar in a child's diet.

Today, most psychiatrists believe that hyperactivity—or ADHD—is hardly a myth. Results of an NIMH study published in 1990 in the *New England Journal of Medicine* traced ADHD to a specific metabolic abnormality in the brain. The use of Ritalin remains controversial, however. Possible side effects include weight loss, a stunting of growth, irritability, upset stomach, insomnia, and mild elevations of blood pressure. But most parents are increasingly willing to try the medication to help their children. Ritalin can keep kids on task during school days, and be discontinued after school, and on weekends and holidays, if side effects become evident. Ritalin won't help all hyperactive children, but because it has been used for fifty years, scientists are more knowledgeable about its long-term effects than most other psychiatric medications.

Feingold's thesis has never been sufficiently proven, though a number of frightened parents bought into the idea wholeheartedly, including Beverly and William M. of Johnstown, Pennsylvania. This entry in Beverly's diary—a letter to her seven-year-old son—illustrates the great resistance to drug therapy and a mother's hope and eventual disappointment:

Nov. 14, 1982

Dear David,

We've had some problems with you & I'm going to write about them so that you will understand some things later in your life.

You were really hyperactive and the hyperactive level rose considerably when you returned to school this year. We took you to the city/county clinic to have you evaluated & you tested out very low—almost dull/normal—mostly because you couldn't sit still or concentrate on what was being said or done.

In fact, they wanted to put you on a drug-management program, but I said, "Absolutely not!" No one was going to give drugs to my child to keep him under control! They argued with me that you'd be better off on drugs, etc. etc. I knew that you were very hard to handle with your incessant tantrums, screaming, constant running to & fro and getting into all kinds of mischief. If it was naughty, you did it, and it didn't seem to matter how many times you got a spanking or how hard we spanked you. You were getting to be more than we could handle & I began to hate to be around you. Each night, I couldn't wait to put my screaming, tantrum-riddled boy to bed & then I would sit dazed for about an hour before I could drag my frazzle-nerved body off to bed. Each day became a loathsome chore to take care of you—I hated it & I hated myself for not wanting to care for you.

Well, in desperation, the therapist suggested we try the Feingold Diet since I was so unalterably opposed to drug-management programs for you. I said I'd do anything for my boy rather than try drugs so we bought the Feingold Diet books, read them, and then stuck to the diet. After four days, the therapist herself couldn't believe the change in you. She even admitted that she thought she had misdiagnosed your problems.

You've been on the diet about five weeks now and it is a pleasure to care for you now. You are obedient and today when it came time to go home from church I was able to keep track of you in the crowded foyer & you followed me out of the church and into the car with no problems. 5 weeks ago I would have had to chase you all over the building & carry you kicking and screaming out into the car.

What made you hyperactive . . . ?

I like you the way you are since you've been on the diet!

We're glad we don't have to put you on the drugs!

Results of the Feingold Diet on David were only briefly sustained. His parents watched helplessly as David's behavior deteriorated, as reflected by this letter from mother to son, three and a half years later:

May 25, 1986

Dear David,

Life has been very difficult for me and for you.

Last summer, you played baseball with East Hills Recreation. It was a terrible experience for me because you used the bat as a weapon & most of the mothers talked unkindly to me about you. I felt terrible. You did a lot of fighting at school, also. I've felt so badly about your behavior that I didn't write anything in this journal for a long time . . .

In the early 1970s, Bill Pelham decided that if he was to succeed in his mission, he would have to know a great deal about Ritalin. "So I spent a lot of time studying medication. The more I studied the data, the more it became clear that medication didn't look all that bad for some kids. I concluded that if we combined medication and behavior management, we might get the best results of all."

Pelham was critical of the hit-or-miss process of selecting specific psychiatric medications for children. "Typically, a doctor decides what medication would be good, and he writes a prescription. A week later, the parent might call or the physician will contact the parent and say, 'How's Johnny doing?' That's the only information transferred between the person writing the prescription and the people watching the kid when he's medicated—unless something goes wrong."

Dosage is also hit-or-miss. Normally doctors will guesstimate, based upon a patient's size, age, and medical history. A process of adjustment or "fine-tuning" takes place, until an acceptable "trough" (maximum medication safely processed in the patient's bloodstream) level is determined. This was precisely the way in which Meggan Scanlon received lithium during her first Western Psych admission, lithium and Tegratol for her second admission, and lithium, Tegratol, and Clonipine while she was seeing Kenneth Stanko.

Thus Pelham's mission changed. Instead of demonstrating that drugs were not as effective as behavioral management, he decided to develop a more scientific way of selecting and using medication through an all-intensive behavioral management program. Over a period of thirteen years, first at the University of Florida and then at Western Psych, Pelham established an eight-week summer program, modeled like a day camp, for ADHD kids, based upon a point system. "Kids who behave and follow instructions get points. They do bad things, they lose points. At the end of the day—or week—they trade their points in for privileges, activities, gifts at the school store."

The difference between Pelham's program and other behavioral management efforts is the frequency and intensity with which kids are evaluated. Instead of limiting the point system to the classroom or predesignated activities, kids are evaluated unyieldingly throughout the day. Five counselors, usually graduate students recruited from universities throughout the U.S., are assigned to one of eight groups of twelve ADHD kids. One counselor, armed with pencil and clipboard, announces a "point check"—in which points are given or taken away—every twenty minutes. This system is in effect during softball and soccer games, as well as in art and literature classes.

Pelham believed that mentally ill kids in general and ADHD children specifically are often ostracized by siblings and peers for poor performance in athletics and lack of social skills. At Pelham's school, counselors score children as avidly in recreational activities as in the classroom. At a softball game, counselors awarded points not only when kids caught a ball or got a hit, but also when they could recite the vital statistics—"What's the inning? How many outs? What's the score?"

"Playing baseball actually demands a tremendous amount of attention," Pelham says. "The social consequences are terrible if, for example, the other team wins the game because you are facing the wrong way when the ball is hit and it goes over your head."

Throughout the day, points are awarded when kids disagree but settle their differences calmly, through discussion and negotiation; points are taken away when kids yell, curse, throw punches, and so on. Quite literally, a child is rated for every conceivable educational, recreational, artistic, or social interaction. How does this intensive behavioral management program relate to the use of Ritalin? Each kid is evaluated during the eight weeks under four separate drug-related scenarios. The first two weeks none of the kids are given any drugs at all. Points are awarded and taken away. If the behavioral management/point system seems to be successful, then a kid might never receive Ritalin—or any other medication. If the point system is ineffective, then kids are given medication—a lower dose, a higher dose, or a placebo, in weekly increments—without knowing what they are receiving. Behaviors are observed and evaluated under each of these circumstances, and the information fed into the camp computer. At the end of the summer, Pelham will be able to demonstrate if and under what circumstances Ritalin is helpful for each individual patient.

As valuable as this information may be to parents and doctors, Pelham stresses that one eight-week summer program is not enough for severe and chronic ADHD kids. "Response to medication doesn't stay the same over the years. So a person should have a repeated assessment. Another thing is, kids can learn a lot about the proper behavior in one summer and forget everything in the intervening nine months, if they aren't involved in ongoing treatment." Pelham conducts a weekend program for kids during the school year, while one night a week during the summer, parents attend a three-hour workshop to learn the point system and how to advantageously enforce it for the child back home.

Although Pelham's is not the definitive study of medication and ADHD—the culmination of his mission—it is a logical and efficient method of maximizing what is currently the only existing and relatively safe therapeutic intervention for chronic and severe ADHD kids. On the surface, the camp sounds expensive: about $250 per day, per child. But compare that to similar inpatient programs at Western Psych and other hospitals in the U.S. with a daily rate of $1,400. Experts predict that this kind of "day treatment" program will become increasingly popular. It is possible that Meggan Scanlon did not need to be admitted to Western Psych for seven months, for instance; Elizabeth and Tom might have managed her at home if such a program had been available.

Pelham's day camp and concept have fostered similar programs through-out the U.S., including a year-round school founded by a former student in Irvine, California.

During my periodic observation at Pelham's ADHD program, held coincidentally at Winchester Thurston, I was surprised and frightened by the insistent wildness and lack of control exhibited by ADHD kids. I had interviewed ADHD experts and listened to their stories—and believed them. Yet the reality of ADHD was startling. If the children could not be controlled by full-time, trained counselors, I began to understand the frustrations of parents home alone with an ADHD child. I was also struck by how closely ADHD kids displayed behaviors mirroring Tom's and Elizabeth's descriptions of how Meggan acted at home.

THE FIVE COUNSELORS responsible for one of the adolescent groups supervised by Betsy Hosa, a Pelham protégée, usher their charges into a classroom at Winchester one morning, then settle down in the corridor for their daily staff meeting. No sooner does the meeting begin than Jerry, a wiry, brown-haired twelve-year-old, is dragged from the class-room by one of the teachers, kicking and screaming, and put in a "time-out" in the corner.

The moment the teacher returns to the classroom, Jerry begins punching the wall with his fist. After a few minutes, punching is not enough, so he begins to kick and bang his head. Although they have been trying to ignore the commotion and maintain a discussion, Hosa relents and assigns Cheryl, a senior from Purdue University, to calm and supervise Jerry. The moment Cheryl returns to the group, Jerry suddenly streaks down the hall and charges into the classroom, screaming ob-scenities.

Hosa sends Stan, a tall graduate student from Yale, to replace Cheryl. Jerry has no respect for Stan, either. At the earliest oppor-tunity, he breaks away and attempts to return to the classroom through the rear door. Stan dashes after Jerry, grabs him, and pushes him into a corner, blocking his way, until he promises not to move. Stan eventually permits Jerry to return to the classroom, but minutes later, Jerry is ejected once again. Stan cannot control the situation, even though he and Cheryl have deducted hundreds of points from Jerry's total. Jerry is screaming, kicking, his arms flailing uncontrollably. Stan pins Jerry to the floor; Jerry screams louder. Hosa tells Stan to take Jerry to the "principal" (Pelham) for more serious disciplinary action.

Now Alan takes Jerry's place in the time-out corner in the corridor. Spotting a light switch, he begins to flick it on and off. The hallway is dark, bright, dark. Stan deducts points until Alan calms down. A few minutes later, Alan is making loud and disgusting noises, echoing up and down the hallway. He takes his shoes off and starts pounding them on the floor. "Hey, Stan," Alan screams, "quit shitting in your pants."

The classroom door is opened and another boy is ejected. It is not clear what is happening in the classroom, but it sounds like a riot has been ignited. The kids are yelling, "Fuck you; suck shit." The counselors are uncomfortable and embarrassed, shaking their heads and muttering, "This has not been a very good day."

One of the reasons I felt the behavioral milieu was not always effective on 3 West was because it was too complicated, especially for some of the kids of lower intelligence or with learning disabilities. To understand the rules, punishments, and rewards, patients were asked to digest a sixteen-page typewritten booklet written in vague and imprecise language, making it difficult for even the brightest patients to comprehend what was expected of them.

Similarly, Pelham's point system was complicated—even for the counselors. One morning I overheard a brief conversation concerning how many points to take away from Jerry because of his use of the term "It sucks." If Jerry said "It sucks" in a moderated voice then, under Pelham's point system, the phrase would constitute "complaining," which represents a smaller deduction of points. But if Jerry said "It sucks" in a loud or aggressive manner, it would constitute "negative interaction" which, said one counselor, is "higher in the hierarchy of point penalties than complaining."

As it turns out, Jerry made it through the eight-week treatment program, but Pelham admits that minimal progress was made in preparing him for the outside world. Jerry is an ideal example of the challenges inherent in coping with severe mental illness. He has been taking Ritalin and has been given special treatment for three summers in

Pelham's program—and he has not made significant progress. Later in the summer, Pelham and Hosa designed an even more intensive behavior modification program for Jerry, but it did not help to curb his behavior. In the not-too-distant future, Jerry may begin to resist taking medication, which will undoubtedly trigger even more oppositional behavior. The only hope for Jerry and perhaps also for Meggan Scanlon is that their ADHD (if ADHD is indeed Meggan's problem) will dissipate. "Many times ADHD goes away—disappears—as adolescents near adulthood," says Pelham. "But we don't know when or why this happens."

17

BECAUSE OF INSURANCE limitations, Meggan cannot stay at Western Psych for any more than thirty-five days—with three admissions per year. There are few options remaining, none of which seems workable. Technically, Meggan can return home, but Tom and Elizabeth have decided that this is unacceptable. They are ready to relinquish custody, *if* CYS and Orphan's Court will allow such an action. Even if relinquishment is permitted, who will guarantee that Meggan is placed in a desirable facility? For that matter, does a desirable facility exist for Meggan Scanlon? And where does Meggan live until she can be placed there? Time is running out for Tom and Elizabeth. The only interim solution is a transfer to Mayview, which would be inappropriate. But Dr. Boris has the power and the influence to find Meggan a bed there, at least temporarily.

YOU LOOK GOOD in black," Tom Scanlon tells Debbie Rubin, as he settles into his seat, opposite her desk. Rubin smiles and swivels back and forth in her chair. In addition to her black suit, she is wearing new red shoes. I know they are new because I have never seen them before, and over the past year, I have been in a position to notice a great variety of Debbie Rubin's shoes. From my vantage point across the room, behind Debbie and opposite Tom and Elizabeth, I have noted that Debbie hides her feet under her desk and slips off her shoes whenever her therapy sessions become difficult. When she turns toward the Scanlons, her face will remain impassive despite the intensity of the experience, the sadness or confrontation which she will sometimes precipitate, but her toes are preoccupied—twirling, dangling, tangoing with her shoes.

Rubin is forty years old. She has an eight-year-old son whose photograph sits in a gold and silver frame on her desk; her husband is a cardiologist at a large community hospital two miles from campus. Rubin was born and educated in Pittsburgh, but a dozen years ago moved with her husband to Boston, where she first worked as a psychiatric social worker. Following her husband back to Pittsburgh, she was offered a position on 3 West. Her father had been a social worker at Western Psych; he retired in 1976 as director of the Social Work Department.

Elizabeth initiates the discussion by pointing out that Meggan continues to insist she is going home after her discharge from Western Psych. If they cannot get her into a special school or group or foster home through CYS in Pittsburgh, however, Elizabeth is contemplating a move to North Carolina, where her sister lives and where services for emotionally disturbed children are more readily available.

Suddenly, Elizabeth points her finger and speaks to Debbie Rubin accusingly. "If you make me take Meggan back home this time, I swear to God . . ." She pauses and takes a deep breath. "I won't take her back home—no matter what."

Elizabeth takes a deep breath and begins again, taking a different tack. She says that it is becoming increasingly important to her that Meggan learn to achieve something—*anything*—at school, *any school.* "I am not looking for too much. I don't need her to become President of the United States or a brain surgeon. But she used to have such energy! At North Country, she plugged into that energy. She learned to ice-skate—and she absolutely loved to ski. She got into batik. She made me a dumb little fish. It wasn't anything, but it was so neat.

"Meggan is a terrific student. If you were a teacher, you would kill for a student like my daughter. She's creative, she's exciting—she's weird. She's always been appreciated more by adults than by the kids her own age, and she usually hooked herself into her favorite teacher. The kids thought she was strange. Well, for God's sake, I knew more than anyone how strange and weird she was. But I have always fought for her right to be different." Now tears are rolling down Elizabeth's cheeks. "Meggan is telling people on the unit that she is a vampire. This is her way of acknowledging that she will be forever different."

Debbie Rubin passes a box of Kleenex. Elizabeth nods appreciatively and dabs her eyes.

"And when is the worst possible time in life to feel different?" Rubin asks.

"When you are a teenager."

"What do you think Meggan is going to say when she learns that she is really not coming home—that your willingness to relinquish your parental rights is for real?"

"I know that Meggan knows that I love her. And that is a heck of a big step from one generation to another because when I was her age, my mother never made me feel that way. But," Elizabeth adds, "your question is only theoretical. I don't have any confidence that she is not going to come home—despite what you say." Once again, Elizabeth looks accusingly at Debbie Rubin.

"I don't know what to say to you about sending Meggan to Mayview or anywhere else," says Rubin. "I don't have the answers right now. We have to play a waiting game. We have to sit back and see what will happen. There are many options, thanks to Ken Stanko."

Dr. Stanko's contact with the CYS supervisor last month had been effective in setting the wheels of relinquishment in motion. Debbie Rubin had been skeptical when she learned that Stanko had received encouragement from CYS. Based upon her years of contact with the organization, the likelihood that CYS would willingly help the middle-class, well-insured Scanlon family was very low. Probably the supervisor with whom Stanko consulted was being polite to the naive private practitioner, she had then speculated, "although miracles do tend to happen at CYS, every few hundred years." But when Meggan returned to 3 West, Rubin telephoned CYS to investigate. She was surprised and delighted to discover that Meggan Scanlon's case had been officially opened—a vital first step. But this positive turn of events had no effect on the Scanlons, already stung and paranoid with a history of fifteen years of ideas and promises by doctors and an irresponsive system. Elizabeth began describing the joyous state of their lives with Meggan out of the house. "We have a wonderful family when the three of us—me and Tom and Doug—are together. Doug thinks I am a great mother."

"Doug and I have never been closer," says Tom.

"He's our pride and joy. He gets into trouble from time to time, but he tells us the truth. Meg insults us."

"What does it take to convince people to get her off the streets?" Tom asks. "Does she need to be gang-raped? Should we let her kill someone with a car?"

"If we had enough money our problems would be solved," said Elizabeth. "But there's nothing left; no college money, no savings. It all went to Meggan's therapists and her private schools." The Scanlons are $42,000 in debt, "completely at risk every day of our lives."

Tom sighs, squirms, and turns to face the wall. "I have to abandon my daughter in order to receive public services? I guess I haven't paid my taxes all these years."

"I can't understand why you refuse to refer her to Mayview," Elizabeth says to Debbie Rubin.

"It is not clear to me that Meggan is not going to Mayview," Rubin replies calmly.

"What I have always hoped is that someone would take her away from us and take care of her," says Elizabeth. "But after North Country, I wished she was dead." She pauses to snatch another Kleenex and wipe her eyes.

"In lieu of that—I mean instead of killing her, which is what I really want to do—I have decided to leave. To leave Tom, to leave Meggan, to leave Doug—everybody. It's not pretty, it's not right, but that's all there is. I have begged for help, I have demanded help. But I can't do it anymore. I can't go on. I'm leaving home."

"I have been watching you out of the corner of my eye," Debbie says to Tom. "What are you thinking?"

"I am sitting here listening to my death sentence," he replies.

"Yours or Meggan's?"

"If Meggan comes home, Elizabeth will leave me. I feel like someone is passing a life sentence over me for a crime I did not commit."

Tom remembers the last time Elizabeth left him—an incident precipitated by the same question with which they are attempting to deal today: what to do with Meggan? It had occurred the summer following her expulsion from North Country. Because of continued warfare between the two children, Doug and Meggan could not be at home at the same time, and the Scanlons had exhausted their pool of babysitters willing to go head-to-head with Meggan. Because Doug was younger, it was easier to find child care for him outside the home, although at thirteen, he had had enough.

"One afternoon, Douglas and I were having a rather loud discussion about the problem," said Elizabeth. "I was upset and he was upset and we weren't coming to any good conclusions. Meggan suddenly started telling me how I should have handled the situation."

Elizabeth had always known deep in her heart that sooner or later she would reach a point of no return—a moment in time when her daughter's unyielding assaults upon her would force her either to lose her mind entirely or to flee. Meggan had always been able to hurt her by instinctively saying things to which Elizabeth was most sensitive. "I've talked to other mothers with kids like Meggan. They all relate the same kind of thing. Sometimes you know damn well you did wrong, but it's extraordinarily painful to listen to." Ordinarily Elizabeth would have fought back, or locked herself in her room. But Meggan had picked the absolute worst moment to launch an attack. "I left the house and moved in with a girlfriend."

Although Tom understood that Elizabeth had reached a breaking point—and needed respite from Meggan—the days he remained alone as a single parent had been devastating. "There were days when I went to work and could barely function. The night that Elizabeth left I just sat and cried the whole night. Meggan made fun of me. She said, 'You're acting like a jerk. She'll be back. What are you worried about?' Doug was as upset as I was. He went into his room and cried. I sat on the bed and cried with him. Meg went out and chose not to come home until midnight without telling me where she was going. I could have just killed her." Tom snaps a Kleenex from the box and dabs the tears from his eyes. He buries his face in his hands.

"I simply have to get away because I get afraid that I'm just going to die, that this situation with Meggan is going to kill me, that she is killing my soul," says Elizabeth. "It sounds really awful. I feel helpless and out of control. I can barely talk when Meggan is home, because I don't have anything to offer her anymore. I visualize myself as one of the shadows on the street after the bombing of Nagasaki and Hiroshima. I saw the pictures of those people who were just mere shadows on the pavement. That's how empty I felt when I had left Tom. I felt like there was nothing there. I had no presence. I was a shadow on the pavement. I had to get out.

"My best friend is divorced. She's been on her own for years. She goes home every night to a quiet apartment and plays whatever she wants on the radio—something wonderful. You go over there and it's quiet. Oh my God! I can remember going to see her at lunch and crying and saying, 'I want your life. I just want your whole life. I'll give up everything else. Let me have it.' It's becoming harder and harder to function, to get through the day. I have to get . . ." She searches for the words, but Rubin finds them:

"You have to get away from Meggan—your daughter."

"That's right."

"And you are willing to sacrifice your relationship with Tom?"

"I will never sacrifice my relationship with Tom. But don't you see? My feeling for Tom is deep inside of me, and it will never go away. Practically, I can live without him."

"But can Tom live without being with you?"

"No, he can't."

"So what is going to happen to Tom if you leave?"

"What is going to happen to me," asks Elizabeth, "if I stay?"

Debbie Rubin's shoes have been on and off four times in the past ten minutes. Her voice becomes high-pitched during such tense moments, and she has the tendency to press her chin on her fist and mumble, forcing Tom to lean forward. "I can't hear you," he says.

"The sad part about all of this," says Rubin, repeating herself, "is that your guilt over giving up Meggan is not going to go away even if you are successful in placing her somewhere. You will both always feel like beasts."

"She makes me feel like a hostage," says Elizabeth. "Any moment, she is going to take her hot poker out and burn me again. I can't explain it to people. She makes me feel like a battered wife. I can't deal with her. I can't deal with a child who relishes my hurt. The more that I hurt, the happier she is. There ought to be shelters for battered mothers to protect them from their children. I cannot continually be terrorized by a child. The cost is too high."

"So listen to me," says Debbie Rubin. "I think that the one person who has gotten you through all of this is Tom."

"That's absolutely true," says Elizabeth.

"But you want to leave him?"

"Tom can't protect me from her. He wants to, but he can't." Elizabeth raises her voice. "I won't look for a new husband, and he won't be looking for a new wife. I will be with him in heart and spirit for the rest of my life."

She is sobbing hysterically. She begins to choke. The four of us sit in silence while she calms herself. "Life wasn't really supposed to be this hard. It really wasn't," she finally says.

"We will work together and do all we can to accomplish your objectives. We will make phone calls to anyone who will listen. We will fight the fight together," Rubin tells them.

"What kind of time frame are we talking until you send her home?" Tom asks abruptly.

Rubin remains calm, but she is clearly perplexed. "I keep trying to tell you that I don't know that we are going to send her home. We are talking the worst-case scenario—home. We know that we can keep her for another month—we have our ways to do that, to sway the insurance company. And there's a chance to get her into Mayview for anywhere from three to nine months. And then maybe group homes."

Tom's face is red and wet. His voice is choked and weak. "For Godsakes, Debbie, get her in there—to Mayview. Get her anywhere. Just for a while. Please."

"Maybe we should sell the house and move into an apartment, take all the money that's left and send her to school for one more year," says Elizabeth.

"I'll do that, happily," says Tom. "I'll do anything," he adds.

Now Tom is sobbing. Elizabeth is crying quietly. Debbie Rubin watches them both, playing with her shoes and pressing her fist into her face.

Tom says, "I have never been happier in my life than I have been with Elizabeth."

"Then you have to fight for what you want, Tom," Debbie Rubin says.

"I'm trying," says Tom. "I am fighting with all my power."

"There's a limit to my strength," says Elizabeth. "I must have peace."

"How peaceful will it be without Tom?"

"The only other solution that I can think of is suicide," says Elizabeth.

With the exception of playing with her shoes, Debbie Rubin has skillfully led the session without exhibiting a great deal of emotion. She has been warm, attentive, and responsive. Even now, Rubin does not change her expression. She maintains eye contact with the distraught mother. Rubin knows that suicide is not a new idea for Elizabeth, for she has previously admitted to Debbie that she considers death a viable option to living with Meggan. But this time, she has added another frightening wrinkle to her destructive scenario.

"You would leave Tom and Doug with that legacy of suicide?" Rubin asks her.

"No," says Elizabeth calmly. "My new idea is that we will all three make the choice of going together."

18

THE TORMENT AND desperation Elizabeth and Tom demonstrated during family therapy convinced Debbie Rubin and Dr. Boris to find a way of keeping Meggan on 3 West as long as possible, hoping that something good would happen for the family. Over the previous weeks, Ritalin had proven effective for Meggan, whose attention span in the 3 West school had improved, and she seemed less irritable. But Ritalin was a short-term medication, while desipramine, a more sophisticated stimulant, could theoretically be effective twenty-four hours a day. Thus, Dr. Boris launched a desipramine trial on Meggan, beginning with a small dose and gradually adding more each day. Because of the possibility of toxic side effects, medical monitoring and periodic blood tests were important, thereby providing Dr. Boris with a legitimate reason—at least, enough of one to satisfy the insurance company—to keep Meggan hospitalized.

The danger of desipramine had partially justified extending Meggan's admission, but the situation nevertheless reflects the wasteful and ludicrous way in which medical professionals are forced to function because of lack of alternative facilities and programs. Meggan's desipramine trial could have been maintained on an outpatient basis or in a school setting where she could be closely observed, as William

Pelham has demonstrated at his ADHD camp. Her counselors and teachers could effectively report and compute her behaviors.

The Scanlons were willing to allow Meggan to return home while the trial was in effect and while they were awaiting CYS's decision as to what—if anything—should be done with Meggan. But such largess might send the wrong message. Taking her out of the hospital and bringing her back home would signify improvement, thus leading to the assumption that institutionalization was unnecessary. It was in Tom and Elizabeth's best interest to see Meggan deteriorate.

Over and above their worries concerning CYS's final decision, the Scanlons were also concerned about where Meggan might be placed, *if* she were placed at all. There were a number of residential treatment centers within a hundred-mile radius, but at the moment none had openings. Ideally, the Scanlons would want Meggan as close as possible so that they could visit her regularly; Meggan could even come home on weekends sometimes. But if they refused an admission for Meggan she could lose priority and be shuffled to the bottom of the list. There might never be another opportunity for placement—unless precipitated by a crisis. They were prepared to agree to anything.

Linda Steen, the single parent from Memphis who relinquished custody of her daughter, Marney, had been in a similar situation. Because she felt pressured to find a place for her daughter after having gone through a long judicial ordeal, she agreed to a placement even though it forced her to travel 250 miles round-trip each weekend. But compared to many of the most seriously disturbed children and their families in the U.S., Ms. Steen and Marney are fortunate, as a disturbing and revealing study conducted by the National Mental Health Association, called "The Invisible Children" Project, demonstrates.

According to the NMHA, which collected data from thirty-seven states, more than 4,000 children with severe mental health problems had been placed in out-of-state facilities, sometimes thousands of miles from home, at an estimated annual cost of $215 million. In Maryland alone in 1989, 680 children were sent to out-of-state residential treatment centers as far away as Vermont and Florida. These isolated kids, together with approximately 25,000 children in state hospitals, often in remote locations, foster children, and kids in juvenile justice facilities, bring the total number to 600,000 children in out-of-home placement in 1991 at a combined federal and state cost of $9 billion.

Although the number of children with mental health problems in out-of-state placement is growing, a few innovators have been successfully fighting the trend, with the state of Alaska leading the way. The Alaskan Youth Initiative (AYI) is the creation of John VanDenBerg, a transplanted Kansan, working as a consultant for the Alaskan Departments of Education and of Health and Social Services.

In the early 1980s, VanDenBerg told me, Alaska lost a great deal of revenue, due to declining oil prices. To save money, state officials decided to repatriate Alaska's "invisible children," many of whom had been in out of state placement for half of their lives. A second, equally important objective was to prevent other children and adolescents from being transferred out of state in the process.

VanDenBerg, a bearded six-foot-five, 275-pound giant, was given this assignment through funding from the NIMH's CASSP. Although the various departments responsible for kids with mental health problems were located in the same office building, officials didn't communicate, didn't even know one another, which wasn't surprising to VanDenBerg, who had served the previous half dozen years at a residential treatment center. VanDenBerg introduced a number of revolutionary yet logical concepts, ideas that were not necessarily new but that had never been put together and utilized on such a large scale.

He convinced his superiors (with the approval of the governor) to use money being spent on out-of-state placement—about $72,000 annually—to design and implement therapeutic programs specifically for each child, without sending them hundreds or thousands of miles away. This concept of "individualized care" became the cornerstone of AYI, along with "flexible funding." Let the money follow the kids, VanDenBerg explained, "rather than the kids and families being slaves to the money." In other words, in the traditional system, children and adolescents *had* to go to hospitals, group homes, and RTCs—whether or not they were expected to be therapeutic. There was nothing else available. VanDenBerg and his staff could determine how this money was to be used for each child without being bound by a conventional mode of treatment.

VanDenBerg knew, as do most other experts in the mental health world, that treatment of kids with mental health problems is anchored upon a concept that once made sense but is now basically ineffective. "The system does not react to the child—the child and family are forced to adapt to the system." In Alaska, he reversed this devastating direction.

VanDenBerg also instituted a no-rejection policy, another important concept of AYI. As with Daniel and Terri, hospitals and group homes ejected their patients, often in punishment for behaviors which were uncontrollable. But no matter how often and to what ends kids attempted to sabotage the therapy VanDenBerg and his colleagues fashioned for them, they could not engineer their own rejection, thus reinforcing the notion of their unworthiness to themselves and others. The kids would have a constant and uniform team of adults to work with, despite their behavior.

VanDenBerg next designed a plan to help interagency coordination by introducing case managers, a program also stimulated by CASSP grants, to ensure regular communication with everyone on the team, including patient and family. VanDenBerg was flexible and creative in the selection of the case manager—father, uncle, or next-door neighbor, anyone willing to be dedicated and responsible. This was not a system in which the "professional" ruled, although professionals were part of an interdisciplinary team, responsible for designing a workable plan based upon a creative analysis of a child's circumstances and requirements.

VanDenBerg especially remembers the plan created for a bright, articulate sixteen-year-old boy who had been a local high school wrestling star and an honor student until suffering the onset of severe schizophrenia, becoming wildly psychotic almost overnight. Prior to AYI, this young man would have been instantly institutionalized, perhaps for the remainder of his life. The AYI team initiated a many-faceted program.

Respite services were provided for the family, and counseling and support for the siblings so that they could begin to understand and deal with what had suddenly happened to their brother—and why. Because they lived in a relatively isolated area, the parents were transported by air to Anchorage to meet with other families who had schizophrenic children of the same age. "Meanwhile, we looked at his social needs. He had lost his peer group. His friends were gone. His environment had exploded. He had physical needs. He was not getting exercise because he was cooped up at home. The school didn't want him. The teachers were afraid of him. He had become a truly bizarre kid, big and dangerous and vulnerable to explosion."

A specially trained college student was hired to be a "friend." Working together, they were gradually able to venture out of the house and then across the street—and then even to the movies. "One trigger for his psychosis was contact with females who might be perceived as flirtatious. The team arranged a series of social situations allowing him to be around girls in a totally benign way." A certified special education teacher was hired to work with the boy individually, at the local school, so that he would have contact with his peers. An immediate evacuation program was designed so that his classroom would change from school to home, literally within a few minutes of onset of psychosis. Gradually, he was introduced into regular classes. Later, the team employed the owner of a local store to give the boy a job. A psychiatrist from Seattle specializing in schizophrenia was hired to work with the boy's therapist as a consultant. "The entire package started to click," said VanDenBerg, "and the last I heard, this boy was in his second year of junior college. He's been driving a car; new friends have come into the picture. He has started dating.

"So here's a kid with a biologically-based brain disease. He is still under psychiatric care, takes medications—and is most definitely vulnerable to relapse. But right now, he's on his own. This was a surefire candidate for out-of-state care until eighteen, at which point he would have been transferred into the adult system, a ward of the state for the rest of his life. His schizophrenia has not been cured, but as of six months ago he had gone over a year without a psychotic episode. And he was not in a padded environment—he was in college." VanDenBerg and a number of other mental health experts do not advocate the elimination of hospitalization and psychiatric treatment—on the contrary. But by relying wholly upon institutionalization, medication, and talk therapy, we are arbitrarily eliminating a vast array of other options.

John Burchard, former director of Vermont's Department of Mental Health and currently a professor of psychology at the University of

Vermont, was sent to Alaska by CASSP, along with his wife, Sara Burchard, also a University of Vermont psychologist, to initiate an "independent review" of AYI's individualized care. Over a two-month period, the Burchards conducted seventy-five personal interviews focusing upon a random sample of eleven of the seventy-eight children initially enrolled in AYI.

They met seventeen-year-old Jim, classified as emotionally disturbed and learning-disabled, who had been abandoned by his mother and physically and sexually abused by his father. When transferred into AYI at fourteen, he had been in eleven placements, including two in a psychiatric hospital, was functioning at a fourth-grade level, and was described as "an effeminate, artsy, engaging transvestite, who cross-dressed and sought indiscriminate sex with older men."

AYI placed Jim in a carefully selected foster home with a couple who were experienced parents, committed to supporting rather than fighting Jim's sexual preference. Weekly therapy was introduced with a gay therapist, along with family therapy. Meanwhile, the foster parents attended gay dances with Jim, while providing training and education concerning health and safety. Through newspaper advertisements, fliers, and networking with school counselors, his foster mother initiated an adolescent gay support group. She helped him seek future opportunities in cosmetology, modeling, and fashion. Jim had run away from this foster home ten times during the first three months of placement, but from the moment this new approach was introduced "until the day Jim left home for good, eighteen months later, he did not run away again," the Burchards stated. Jim's behavior has been erratic and promiscuous since he left AYI, but he has gradually matured and stabilized, returning to school and holding down a steady job. It is important to point out that foster-parenting in this particular theater is a full-time job, which is how the AYI specialized foster parents were paid, as much as $25,000 annually.

The Burchards were also impressed with Mary, seventeen, who had had a similarly traumatic childhood of violent sexual and physical abuse by parents and foster parents and had been in fourteen residential placements. She had demonstrated increasingly severe behavioral problems, including stealing, sexual promiscuity and sexually provocative behavior, self-abusive behaviors, suicide attempts, expressions of homicidal intent, and drug abuse. Although psychiatrists had recommended long-term highly restrictive inpatient care, Mary became pregnant and was placed by AYI in foster care "with a young, professionally trained couple who had a very young child of their own.

"After six months," the Burchards observed, "Mary's attitude and behavior had changed completely. She was off drugs, dressed well, had positive emotions, and acted responsibly. She has reportedly done a magnificent job gaining parenting skills by observing the other mother and child and attending parenting classes. She is very caring for her baby and has developed respect for herself. Mary obtained her GED in the spring and gave the commencement address. She was working part time in the community, had visited with her relatives in her tribal village, and at the time of this review, was making plans to enter college in the fall."

Despite the Burchards' careful study, most experts agree that such anecdotal evidence is inconclusive. The few "controlled" studies of programs similar to VanDenBerg's individualized care concept indicate favorable but modest results. But although it cannot yet be scientifically demonstrated, it is evident that the odds against the eleven adolescents the Burchards studied who were breaking free from the traditional institutionalization and establishing a normalized life pattern, even for the brief periods reported in this study, were monumentally against them. And yet, these kids had at least temporarily succeeded through AYI. Daniel had never had the opportunity to succeed at anything.

"We went five years without sending a kid out of state," VanDenBerg said, "and one hundred twenty-eight kids were returned home during that time." Suicide attempts had virtually been eliminated, as had criminal incidents. The first eighteen kids had attempted suicide nineteen times in the six months prior to AYI—but made no attempts for the first six months in AYI. At the end of the first year, the average cost in "individualized care" situations had been reduced to $40,000 from an annual average out-of-state budget of $72,000. "The last thing we need is more money," VanDenBerg told me. "What we need is to learn how to spend the money we have more intelligently."

Many professionals wince at VanDenBerg's cavalier dismissal of additional funding, but his pronouncement symbolizes the importance of doing things differently. Individualized care is a radical alternative for worst-case kids, but there are other, less expensive utilitarian community-based programs based upon the idea of "family preservation" that may be effective under circumstances which vary in intensity.

"Family preservation refers to time-limited intensive interventions offered to a family with a child facing imminent removal from his or her own (or foster or adoptive) family," writes Jane Knitzer, author of *Unclaimed Children*. "Unlike many traditional mental health and child welfare services, where different staff and sometimes even different agencies are assigned to the parent and child, the family preservation therapist works with the entire family. Rather than require that the clients go to an office, in this service, the therapist goes to where the client is, and at the client's convenience."

Providing help on the family's own turf, "the therapist can learn much more in a short time about a family" while reinforcing "the notion that the family is in charge. During the early weeks, the therapist is involved with the family face-to-face . . . up to twenty hours." Instead of breaking up the family to provide children with essential mental health services (or protection), the system dedicates itself to finding a way of accomplishing those objectives while keeping the family intact.

Although there are a number of model programs, one of the most prominent is Homebuilders in Tacoma, Washington, established in 1974. Founders Jill Kinney and David Haapla decided to initiate home-based services at a moment of crisis—the point at which the child was in danger of being removed from the family. By intervening at the exact moment of crisis, a great deal of positive change could be accomplished in a short and intensive time frame.

Geared to react within twenty-four hours, experienced counselors may actually bring sleeping bags to the home and move in with the family, working with each family member until the crisis has passed. For the Scanlons, it might have been the night Meggan stole the family car or the day she returned home from North Country School after trashing the artists' cabin. The Homebuilders staff, mostly master's degree social workers, will prepare themselves for interventions of a month or more. Interventions average about ten hours a week.

Family preservation is not a stick-in-the-mud concept; counselors do not sit in the family living room and "shrink" mom, dad, and kids. They attempt to assess the family's problems, devise mutually agreeable solutions, and help the family attain them. Sometimes the solutions are simple and inexpensive, such as buying a single mother a washer and dryer so that she doesn't have to drag her autistic child to the Laundromat, or helping a family move out of the ghetto and into a better neighborhood by driving them around until they find a suitable apartment. Sometimes the problems are much more difficult, with parents addicted to drugs and alcohol and the children at war with one another or out on the streets scrounging for food. Finding ways to keep mother, father, and children together and enhancing their life quality by devoting a short, intense period of time to their needs, while arranging for ongoing medical and psychological support, is the ultimate objective.

As VanDenBerg indicated, such approaches can not only be effective, but also economical. According to the Edna McConnell Foundation, the average cost of group home placement is $22,400 per child. An episode of acute psychiatric hospitalization costs $45,000; long-term residential psychiatric treatment averages $103,000. The report states: "In Washington, three Homebuilders' therapists can avoid placement for about sixty children in the course of a year. The three therapists cost Homebuilders $145,000, a sum which could be entirely recaptured if the state avoided only nineteen foster care or seven group home placements. In New York City, where Homebuilders has been operating since 1987, the average cost of family preservation services was $5,000 per child, compared to $13,500 per year in foster care. If the city prevented only sixteen foster care placements, it would save enough to pay for family preservation services for forty children."

19

FAMILY PRESERVATION IS a noble concept, but is it always valid? How does society determine the boundaries between potentially good and irreparably dysfunctional families? At what moment should the idealism of keeping a family intact be abandoned for the sake of the child or the family, as in, say, the Scanlons' situation? Did Tom Scanlon's stoic nature, combined with Elizabeth's moodiness and Meggan's "biological" predisposition toward mental illness, add up to an irreversible "poorness of fit"? And, if so, then why is separating Meggan, Terri, or Daniel from their parents looked upon in some quarters as so terrible? Isn't it possible that separation, at least temporarily, could be exactly the right medicine—especially for Terri and Daniel, whose safety had long been at issue?

Americans will not soon forget the tragedy in New York's Greenwich Village of six-year-old Lisa Steinberg, neglected, abused, and eventually killed by her cocaine-addicted adoptive father. Child welfare officials had been contacted by neighbors and teachers alarmed by the regular commotion in the Steinbergs' apartment and concerned for Lisa's safety, but no one with authority would violate the basic commitment to the family unit and intervene, separating the child and the family and perhaps saving little Lisa's life.

For a while, after reading about Lisa Steinberg's horrible home life and seeing the evidence of such abuse in the kids I met at Western Psych, I felt a growing anger toward their mothers and fathers, many of whom had become parents when they were children themselves.

"Many people think that parents are the evil villains," Debbie Rubin told me once when I mentioned my rage and frustration, "including some of the nurses on this unit who identify and sympathize with the kids against the parents." Indeed, tension between the social workers and the nursing staff, based upon the narrow and conflicting "families" versus "kids" orientation, was often in evidence. Social workers like Debbie Rubin were entangled with the family unit, while nurses bond so strongly with the children that they sometimes begin to investigate ways to separate them from parents and guardians—and take them home themselves.

"I understand this thinking," Rubin told me, "but I don't see how blaming the parent does anything more than make you feel like a superior human being. Blaming the parent doesn't help the situation, doesn't help the kid, doesn't help the mom or dad. It doesn't even make you feel particularly better within yourself to heap responsibility on another faceless human being—and it's not necessarily valid.

"I always start with the assumption that the vast majority of parents do the very best they can. That may be pretty terrible in some situations, but when you come right down to it, parents basically want to straighten out their own lives and improve their behaviors. What will automatically punishing parents by separating them from their kids accomplish? Are you doing a kid a favor by sending him to a group home or residential treatment center? You've seen what's available for Daniel and Terri. Have you come across a group home in which you would be willing to live?

"Nor is it right to tell kids that their parents are bad people. In my experience, eight times out of ten, parents are harder on themselves than they deserve. They will tell me repeatedly everything they have done wrong while raising their child, and why their child's behavior is their fault. Sometimes it's minor stuff, like locking their kids in their room for three hours. Or, 'I sent my son to school when he was only four years old, and that's why he has conduct disorder now.' Sometimes it's also major stuff—mothers and fathers are abusive, neglectful; they take drugs, drink.

"But in their hearts, most moms and dads do not want to hurt their children. They are simply unable to deal with their lives, and because of their weakness and instability, their children get hurt. Yes, I think there are bad parents. There are parents who have done unspeakably horrible things to their kids, but I start with the assumption that parents down deep are well-meaning, because if I approach the situation in any other way, I don't have anywhere to go in my work."

Rubin's views about the potential viability of parents of what one NIMH psychiatrist has referred to as "the damaged generation" are confirmed by child psychologist Robert Friedman, director of the Florida Mental Health Institute and the author of the underlying principles of the family-based movement as outlined in CASSP's "system of care." Friedman views the family as the nucleus of treatment and the essential, unavoidable foundation of a child's life. He maintains that no matter what therapeutic approach may be utilized, effectiveness can only be measured later, after the child is returned to his or her roots.

"The process of taking the child out of his or her environment, putting the child in the hospital for a while, and then returning him home is often referred to as the 'auto mechanic mode' of child mental health. If our car is broken, we take it to the garage so the mechanic will fix it. Although our children cannot be repaired and/or replaced like engines and transmissions, the reality is that most hospitalized kids will be sent home and subsequently expected to function somewhat normally. So it only makes sense to do all we can to work in partnership with parents to assist them in improving their own environment, which may subsequently enable them to improve the quality of their children's existence."

Committing resources to support the family is the only pragmatic approach to the problem. The lasting impact of the family—the true and deep ties of early attachment—will withstand the test of time, sometimes illogically, and often with destructive outcomes. "I know kids who lived with foster parents who have been very kind and caring for long periods of time," Friedman told me. "But as soon as they turned eighteen, what did they do? They ran home immediately. It's inevitable. Oftentimes the staff in hospitals or group homes are in disbelief at this blind and illogical loyalty. 'Why are you going back to these people who mistreated you? Why choose to live with the source of your pain and misery, rather than those who have been so giving and caring?' "

I had been struck by the same surprise and disbelief described by Friedman in conversations with kids at Mayview and Western Psych. The vast majority talked incessantly about returning home, while admitting simultaneously that their parents had harmed them. I remember one conversation with Terri. In all those many months she had lived at Mayview, neither of her parents had ever come to see her—not once. "So why would you want to be with people who don't even care enough about you to visit?"

"That's what everybody always asks me," she admitted. "And it doesn't make any sense, but I can't help what I feel. All I ever think about is being back at home with my father and sisters. I can't think of anything else, even though they ruined my life."

Like Terri, Daniel had lived both at Mayview and at Western Psych, had been in foster care and in three different group homes. In contrast to Terri, whose father has always remained in regular, although often volatile, contact, Daniel's mother had officially relinquished custody, a factor that plagued Daniel perhaps more than anything else in his dismaying and tortured life—and another example of the dominant role of early attachment (his biological father abandoned the family early on and has subsequently died).

Why would his mother sign papers symbolizing such a lack of interest and love, pledging to have nothing to do with him as long as she lived—or at least until he was eighteen? She could not seek him out, talk with him, or identify herself if he approached her, Daniel had been told. This was the punishment levied against her for being such a poor parent. Daniel talked about his mother frequently with periodic spasms of love and an inability to understand the "relinquishment," while displaying a general resentment at her for putting him on this earth and then abandoning him. He called her a drunk, a whore, and a beautiful, wonderful woman. He told stories about seeing her secretly in shopping malls, restaurants, and a skating rink to which his group home took him on Saturdays. In one story, he vividly described how they spotted each other from across the rink and rushed toward one another, like in the movies, with outstretched arms. And then, after embracing, they had skated around, arm-in-arm, for the rest of the evening. They made plans to meet every Wednesday after school, her day off. Initially, I tended to believe this and other adventures Daniel had described to me, only to learn later that most of these stories were wishful dreams.

Daniel had once been considered for adoption by a foster family with whom he lived—until a sudden divorce ended all hopes for being part of a family, the dream he most regularly coveted. When I met him, Daniel frequently showed me a tattered black-and-white photograph of him posing with the pony he was given when he lived with this family. He told me that this foster family came to visit him every other weekend and that he spent Christmas, Thanksgiving, and Easter at their tiny farm. When I asked one of Daniel's caseworkers, I was told that the couple had severed all ties with Daniel once they had returned him.

One of the biggest staff problems was what to do with Daniel during holidays when the facility closed. Most kids actually had parents and could go home for a few days, but Daniel, with his tumultuous history, was pretty much unwanted. There are approximately 25,000 older "special needs" children across the U.S., according to the National Committee on Adoption, many of whom are languishing alone in cold and unfriendly institutions. Usually staff members would share responsibility for Daniel over the holidays, because there was nowhere else to put him. He would be passed around, night after night. Over the Thanksgiving weekend, he might be forced to sleep in three different beds.

THE IDEA OF a public welfare agency successfully separating a child from his or her parents in a city even as large as Pittsburgh (population 350,000) is ludicrous. The way the system is structured actually renders the separation impossible unless the child is immediately eliminated from public welfare rolls, such as Daniel's twin, who was quickly adopted. He disappeared, but four remaining children, a boy and a girl older than Daniel and two younger children, remained in the home. Over the next few years, the two eldest children experienced difficulty with juvenile authorities and were placed in a series of group homes and detention facilities—the same group homes in which Daniel was eventually placed.

Daniel had limited contact with his elder siblings, but he heard about them frequently and was often regarded by staff members as being from the same troublesome mold. Daniel's child advocate attorney, who represented him for the regular court hearings which assessed his progress, had also represented his brother and sister, of whom she was frequently critical. Many group homes conduct joint Saturday-evening outings; Daniel and his elder siblings might often find themselves in the same room together. Daniel's family name was in the phone book; he had copied the addresses and phone numbers of all people with his last name in a little notebook he carried. Daniel was sent a variety of mixed messages. His mother and his siblings were bad people, and he was forbidden to see them, yet he was living within a ten-minute ride from his mother's house and often found himself within shouting distance of his brother and sister.

Daniel and his mom, whom I will call Linda, were finally reunited one Saturday afternoon when Daniel's older brother went into Ward Home illegally and, in an act akin to kidnapping, spirited Daniel off to his mother's house as a kind of peace offering, a way of making up for a series of family arguments precipitated by the brother's conduct—drinking, fighting, law-breaking. Although the incident took the people responsible for Daniel—the folks at Ward Home—by surprise, it was another demonstration of their lack of responsibility in protecting and caring for the kids in their charge. Renewed contact with his mother changed Daniel's life, although it seems to have been more destructive than beneficial.

Linda admits that she had not been a particularly responsible mother, but there were circumstances that explained her actions, if not justifying them. For example, her youngest daughter, Jill, who was then five, was suffering from cancer, receiving weekly treatments of chemotherapy. Without money for day care and an absence of family members to help, Linda was forced to leave her older children alone. Admittedly, she drank excessively, but she was tortured by fear for her daughter's life and crippled by a lack of money. Meanwhile, Daniel was not easy to care for; he hallucinated frequently and acted in a bizarre manner—such as the time in the middle of the night when he crawled out on to the roof of their apartment building and stood there for a long time, threatening to jump.

CYS persuaded her to give up custody of Daniel and his twin by threatening to take away her two younger daughters. After Daniel had been sent to Western Psych and subsequently to Mayview, Linda says she attempted to visit Daniel but doctors did not permit it. She had been told that Daniel would be much better off if he never saw her again. The family complied and signed the necessary papers. Over the next year, with Jill in remission, Linda began putting her life together.

Although she too suffered from severe learning disabilities, Linda returned to school and improved her reading skills. She never completed her high school education, but found regular employment as a maintenance person in a downtown office building. She passed the driver's test to get a license, curtailed her drinking, and eventually remarried. But since relinquishing custody she had lived the life of a fugitive, refusing to give her phone number or address to anyone but her closest friends and relatives. CYS had warned her that if she reverted to her old ways they would return and take her remaining two children away. Linda and her new husband, John, had lived in fear that CYS would devastate their family once again.

Beyond the basic verifiable facts, it is difficult to know how much of her story is true, just as it is difficult to understand CYS's motivations in dividing a family, instead of attempting to provide aid and support at a very difficult time. Clearly, however, Linda is a different person today than she was then, although I had my doubts that she could handle such a challenging and disturbed adolescent as Daniel, as much as she was committed to trying. Daniel experienced a great change in personality and purpose once he was reunited with his mother. Normally somewhat accommodating, he suddenly became obsessed with the idea of resuming life at home, as if the child welfare/mental health world had never intervened.

As far as he was concerned, he would soon be leaving Ward Home to move in with his mother or his grandmother. To him the entire arrangement was a fait accompli; the CYS caseworker, the staff at Ward Home, the mother and grandmother, had already approved the arrangement. In a few days, his life as an orphan would be over, and all the terrible things that had happened to him in the interim would be permanently obliterated. But Daniel was nursing an illusion—at least at that moment. Ward Home would have been relieved to get rid of Daniel, but CYS was totally opposed, and without the agency's cooperation Daniel's hopes were dim.

Reality didn't discourage Daniel's ardor; his anger and insistence increased. He vowed to get even with anyone who took a stand against him. He was especially peeved at his child advocate attorney, Judith Patterson, who seemed reluctant to cooperate on this mission. I was convinced Patterson had been as ineffective and insensitive as CYS, but I was equally pessimistic about the wisdom of a return to the source of his initial trauma, reminding Daniel that he had been abused and neglected the last time he had lived with his mom.

Daniel did not take to that reminder very kindly. He spoke in an eerie and disconcerting manner, a rhythmic, obsessed, robotlike chant in which he became a mechanical Daniel, rather than a real one. "Excuse me, excuse me, may I clarify one point. Now that you've brought that up I would like for you to understand. I was not abused in my house. In no way was I molested or abused. It's all been a mistake. The information is untrue."

"Are you sure?"

"Yes, I'm sure. Who told you I was abused? Who?"

"You did."

"Well, excuse me, excuse me. Let me clarify that point right now. I was mistaken."

"What about the man in the woods?"

"He abused my sister, but not me. I know the truth. It wasn't me."

"What about your brother?"

"My mother told me that all the information about child abuse and sexual abuse is completely untrue. That's how I know. I believe her."

Months later, Daniel and his mother had more honest conversations in which she not only admitted that he had been abused, but described in detail the abuse she had suffered as a child. But during that summer and the autumn that followed, they both put forth a smoke screen of denial concerning the nightmares of his past.

As the days passed, nothing seemed to make much difference to Daniel except for contact with his mother. Interspersed with rages in his room and in the Ward Home corridors were incessant and wrenching outbursts of sorrowful and uncontrolled sobbing, followed by rambling and incomprehensible monologues of how desperately he missed his mother and how much he wanted to be back in her arms. He was inconsolable.

His efforts were not translating into progress because his CYS caseworker and his mother were at odds. Linda would not provide her address and phone number, nor permit the caseworker to interview her husband and children and conduct a home inspection. Frightening memories of CYS's last invasion, when Daniel and his brother had been taken away, were much too vivid in her mind. Unfortunately, John's and Linda's suspicion of CYS and their basic resentment of all authority figures, real or imagined—anyone who might have an impact on their lives—would become increasingly detrimental to Daniel as the weeks and months went by. Meanwhile, CYS was perfectly correct in wanting to be assured that Daniel would be entering a safe environment if he was permitted to visit home, although it was ironic that the organization seemed unconcerned about the suitability of Daniel's environment at Ward Home.

A shaky truce was eventually forged, allowing Daniel's family to visit him once a week at Ward Home. The truce placated everyone temporarily, but it was too little too late for Daniel and his mom. The protracted logjam over home inspection, which continued in the CYS offices where Linda would periodically visit, ranting and raving over past ills while refusing to cooperate, was eventually broken in November when Daniel's fire at Ward Home led to his expulsion and his subsequent suicide ideation.

While Daniel lived at Allegheny Neuropsychiatric Institute, where he was transferred after his suicide threat, an Orphan's Court hearing was held, presided over by a well-meaning but uninformed jurist. The CYS caseworker and attorney presented Daniel's situation in a cold and impassionate manner. Linda in her testimony rambled incomprehensibly about a number of matters, including the evils of CYS and the inadequacy of public transportation preventing her from traveling easily to ANI and Ward Home. It was evident in her remarks that she was overcome with guilt over her actions as a mother. It wasn't clear whether she wanted Daniel back—or really down deep *needed* him to come back—in order to feel better about herself. Linda was an inarticulate and slow-witted person, but she felt sincerely horrible about what had happened to her family and wanted desperately to make up for it in any way possible.

During the hearing, consulting psychiatrist Janice Forrester, who had worked with Daniel over the years, explained Daniel's diagnosis, the root of his problems, and the progress of her treatment. She advised against any reunification in the foreseeable future, unless and until Daniel, his mother, and her husband agreed to undergo intense and regular therapy to help facilitate the transition home. She explained Daniel's learning disabilities, his need for restriction and structure. She stressed that his mother and her husband would have to be trained in behavior modification techniques in order to properly care for Daniel. Otherwise, reunification would be a disaster for both Daniel and his family.

Dr. Forrester's presentation was compassionate, informed, and eminently sensible—the only intelligent aspect of the entire proceeding, as far as I was concerned—and it was completely and immediately ignored. The judge listened impatiently to Linda and respectfully to Dr. Forrester, but his decision was a foregone conclusion. Daniel had been institutionalized for too long, and too many kids were wards of the county these days. Sending a kid back home to a parent who had already relinquished custody was unusual, but nothing was inherently wrong with it. Quickly and imperialistically, he ordered Linda to permit the caseworker, whose name was Joseph Buckley, to inspect her home.

Subsequently, Daniel was transferred to another group home, Holy Family Institute, which was a fast bus ride to his mother's house. After Buckley's inspection, Daniel was to be allowed regular weekend visits which, if successful, could lead to a permanent return home—an event which occurred about eight months later and with very little effort on anyone's part. The irony and the waste were incredible. After investing upwards of $2 million and uncountable man-hours in separating Daniel from his mother and supporting him with psychotherapy, special schools, and group homes, the entire system—judge, CYS social workers, everyone—suddenly forgot the past and ignored the advice of the expert they had subsidized over the preceding four years to guide them.

One might hope that returning to his mother and his roots symbolized a new start for Daniel, but life at home with his family was a disaster. If Daniel had disliked his special school, Craig House, he absolutely abhorred the "mainstream" education he was receiving through the Pittsburgh public school system. "They put me in eleventh grade, because it is age-appropriate, but I don't understand what they are talking about. I feel stupid every time somebody asks me a question. Everything goes over my head," he said.

For a while, his mother was forced to work two jobs in order to manage the extra financial responsibilities that Daniel represented. Eventually, she was able to resign from her second job, but even her full-time evening job left Daniel with hours of uninterrupted, unstructured free time to get into trouble. As Dr. Forrester had warned in court and as I have seen confirmed repeatedly, Daniel is unable to concentrate, to focus upon tasks, and to remember warnings, mistakes, etc., without careful and vigilant supervision twenty-four hours a day.

Daniel had been permitted to move back home with the stipulation that a counselor provide one hour a week of family therapy for three months' duration. In other words, a total of twelve hours were allotted to the entire process of reunification—after eight years of separation, preceded by neglect and abuse—for a boy with severe mental health problems and learning disabilities. Conceivably, Linda might have continued the counseling beyond the three-month limit, but John flatly rejected the idea. He was not particularly enamored of Daniel, whose presence changed the entire balance of the family he had come to rely on.

CYS made Linda Daniel's guardian. The only way to become his mother again was through adoption. Meanwhile, John had no connection to Daniel, except for the fact that they lived in the same house and shared an affection for Linda. It was John, however, who stood in the way of Daniel's transfer into a highly regarded school for special needs children. A prerequisite for admission was an interview with Daniel's family—a request John flatly refused. A visit from a social worker or teacher would have represented another threat to the family and to John's own personal freedom. Such an invasion by another stranger into his household was out of the question. John had always concealed himself from me; each time I visited, he was in the bathroom. Once, he remained in the bathroom for more than an hour until I left.

John and Linda were within their rights. They could determine who entered their home and who didn't. But they will not suffer, nor will

CYS, nor the special school, if Daniel cannot read or write and is not prepared to enter the world at eighteen. Daniel was a victim of Linda's and John's collective eccentricity and paranoia. CYS and the special school could have made an exception considering the unfair circumstances, but no one would bend. Daniel suffered while the wheels of the system's abject incompetence rolled ignorantly onward. Because Daniel, Linda, and John remained together for more than three months, CYS counted their reunification a success.

20

TWO WEEKS AFTER Meggan's desipramine trial began, Elizabeth mentioned to the dean of Village Academy, the private school for learning-disabled kids that Doug attended, that she was hoping to place Meggan at Ridgeview, a highly structured residential group home. Wesley Institute operates both Ridgeview and Village Academy, and early the following week Elizabeth was contacted by Ridgeview's director, who reported a sudden unplanned opening. They would accept Meggan, based upon the dean's recommendation, pending a successful personal interview *and* CYS's agreement, which would be a guarantee of payment. All of this had to be accomplished within a week, for they could not afford to hold the opening any longer.

"It was magic time," Elizabeth told me a couple of weeks later, in a relieved and ebullient state. "Everything we had hoped for was suddenly coming true in a couple of incredible, unbelievable days." I understood the context of the situation, but felt uncomfortable listening to Elizabeth. Here was a woman so frazzled and tortured that she was rejoicing at the probability of ostensibly giving away her daughter.

Ridgeview's willingness to immediately accept Meggan Scanlon provided CYS with the necessary push. The agency agreed to give final approval if the Scanlons agreed to officially relinquish custody by the end of the week. Debbie Rubin was able to schedule a court date two days hence. The Scanlons' exhilaration and trepidation were inescapable. "We were terrified; it was happening so fast. We walked around on air—breathless—the whole week, waiting," said Elizabeth. "Debbie Rubin performed miracles in facilitating the process. We are building a shrine for her."

The court hearing took place at 11:00 A.M.; parental rights were relinquished in three minutes flat. By 1:00 P.M., they parked the family car on the grassy hilltop on which Ridgeview was located in a sparsely populated suburban area approximately thirty miles from Pittsburgh. "It was like dominoes," said Tom. "Each barrier clicking off one by one."

The interview went well. Meggan was quiet and reserved, but the following evening, when Tom went to visit her on 3 West, the impact of what was happening had hit home. "It was the Grand Ambush. 'You can't do this to me; I won't go. You tricked me. Give me another chance. Let me come home.' " Meggan's tantrum did not temper the Scanlons' relief and joy. "It was a miracle," said Tom. "I lay in bed night after night, thinking, 'Sooner or later I will wake up and find out that this is all a dream.' "

THE SUDDEN OPENING at Ridgeview that preceded Meggan Scanlon's unexpected admission came about because of a series of unfortunate incidents confronted by Terri, who had been admitted to Ridgeview after her long ECT trial. Ridgeview was to be Terri's first and most important step away from hospitalization, providing her with a new start in life, forever disconnecting her from both Mayview and Western Psych.

Terri actually did well for the first few weeks (the honeymoon period), but her behavior eventually began to fall apart. As time went by, she began to refuse to eat or drink, according to Terri's Ridgeview therapist. Then she inflicted a series of superficial cuts to her wrist. Dr. Boris had explained to the Ridgeview staff that Terri would test them repeatedly—do everything in her power to sabotage her situation—in order to return to the places she felt safest, Western Psych and/or Mayview, where she could wallow in her own martyred defeat. Terri's therapist tried to be understanding and helpful, but the impact and the trauma of Terri's past seemed inescapable.

During a group therapy session about three months after admission, Terri disclosed a sexually abusive incident precipitated by a relative when she was four years old. She had previously admitted to being abused by various males, but had never implicated her family. It was an emotional breakthrough after all those years of silent denial, but it also unleashed a floodgate of increasingly destructive behaviors. "After this disclosure, she cried, she yelled, she got mad, she paced," said the therapist. "When the caseworker came [by law, the incident had to be reported to CYS for investigation], she hid in her room under her blanket. Had a real hard time talking any more about it."

The decline in Terri's behavior climaxed one evening when she slit her wrist with a sliver of glass she had concealed. Terri had lost so much blood by the time she was discovered in her room that her life was in serious danger. Unconscious, she was rushed to the intensive-care unit of a nearby hospital. Because they were ill-equipped for kids as difficult as Terri, whom they concluded needed constant monitoring and regular psychiatric support, Ridgeview administrators decided not to permit her to return. After two weeks in the hospital, Terri was transferred to a transitional shelter about fifty miles from Pittsburgh from which she immediately bolted with a newfound girlfriend. Later that same day, Terri and her friend, hitchhiking on a nearby highway, were picked up by two men whom she says raped and abandoned them. Frightened and alone, Terri and her friend reported the incident to the police. A week later, Terri was readmitted to Mayview.

But the roller coaster of life seemed to have one more difficult dip remaining for Terri during this traumatic cycle. I once joked with Daniel that he was a jinx to himself. He agreed, laughing, but we both knew that there was a measure of truth in the joke. It sometimes seemed as if anything bad that could conceivably happen in someone's life actually did happen to Daniel—and to Terri. For most other people, when bad things happen, there are support systems to fall back on: family, colleagues, etc. But extensive institutionalization promotes loneliness and aloneness. Terri lacked a trusting, stabilizing force for support in times of ultimate stress.

After about a month at Mayview, Terri's mood began to stabilize. She was improving at a surprisingly rapid rate, without the help of new medication, ECT, or intense therapy. People who had known her for a long time were surprised and pleased by her optimistic outlook toward the future, based upon a revelation that came while in the ICU recovering from the wound she had inflicted upon herself at Ridgeview. Lying in that bed, having momentarily hovered in a state close to death, Terri suddenly realized that she did not want to die. Her life had been unpleasant, choked with pain, disappointment, and confusion, but she had much to live for. If her parents had no use for her, that was okay, for she had loving siblings, including a younger brother and two elder sisters who had pieced their lives together, graduated high school, and joined the Navy. It came to her that if she worked hard and straightened out her life, she could have a real future, like her sisters'. Excitement about becoming a pediatric nurse or attending law school after college bubbled daily from her lips.

Her optimism was suddenly shattered soon after when Terri learned that one of her sisters, whom she sought to emulate, was killed in a shipboard accident. Terri was permitted to return home for the funeral, but back at Mayview the following day she began to inflict cuts and scratches upon herself, the optimism of her revelation fading into the empty and painful past.

LYNN BIEDA had become Meggan Scanlon's therapist at Ridgeview after Terri's departure. "Meggan assumed a superior attitude," Bieda told me soon after Meggan's admission. "None of the kids gave much credence to her constant complaints about her parents, considering the fact that most of them don't even have parents or don't know where their parents are. Meggan claims that she doesn't understand the issues separating her from her parents, and she rattles off her story as if she has read it in a book, with no emotion. Meggan is quite content with being the person she is, which is oppositional, self-centered, manipulative, impulsive. She has all the right social skills, knows the psychological jargon, but has no interest in going past the superficial stuff and getting to the real issues. We're stalemated at the present time."

Meggan expressed her dissatisfaction with Ridgeview, more because of the other residents rather than anything specific about the facility. "It is impossible to get along with the kids here," she told me. "The staff says the kids are tired of me complaining about my parents. I should realize how lucky I am to have parents. Maybe that's true, but I am tired of my parents harping on me. Our last family meeting, they brought up my fetish about cleaning my room in the middle of the night and how I made their lives miserable. Why do they want to keep bringing up this old stuff? I'm sick of it.

"It was much easier to manipulate the staff at Western Psych. If you exhibited good behavior, they let you go home. Like that stupid journal. I wrote down everything they wanted to hear. I could blow them over with my good intentions and my good behavior. And I could stonewall them to death. My parents always fell into my trap.

"One time with Debbie Rubin we were supposed to work out a behavioral contract. I would write down mistakes I made at home and my parents were supposed to write down how they would punish me if I violated the contract and reward me if I held to our agreements. I didn't tell them, but I thought this was a good idea. My parents don't keep their word, but on paper, I could have held them to their promises. I could have said, 'Look what you promised. It's here in black and white.' But I played my game, acted difficult so that I could get the best deal. That's what you're supposed to do in contract negotiations, isn't it? But what happened? Everybody gave up. It was all really a stupid waste. We would have had a written contract, if they would have kept at it. I was just being difficult, as usual, but they caved in.

"It's very different for me here. The kids have all been raped, molested; their parents have died or have committed serious crimes. And then there's me with my history of private schools and a supportive family, and it's like, 'Why do you hate life so much? Look how good you've had it.'

"When I came here the kids told me I have to assume an attitude, be willing to fight. I have to break the rules to get along. Because that's the code—you have to break the rules to gain respect. And you have to be tough. If someone says, 'Shut up, bitch,' you have to say, 'Don't tell me to shut up, bitch.' And then you have to do something more drastic than what they did to you—hit them or poke them. And no matter what they do to you, you have to always force yourself to say, 'You cannot hurt me. I will kill you if you touch me. Stay away.'

"You have to make them so scared that they won't pick on you anymore. That's what you're supposed to do, although I haven't been able to do it. I don't have the attitude that they want me to have, and so I'll never fit in." She looked wistful and smiled. "I would just love to go back to Western Psych where I belong."

Meggan actually adjusted quite well after a few months. Her grades improved and her mood stabilized. One day, without much advance warning, she was removed from Ridgeview, "an unbelievably ironic turn of events," Elizabeth Scanlon told me. Meggan was placed by CYS with a foster family in the same neighborhood as the Scanlons live, thus completing a $500,000 journey, ending back where it all started a little more than two years ago.

At about the same time Meggan was moved back into her old neighborhood, Tom Scanlon began experiencing massive anxiety attacks, periods of severe shortness of breath, and an inability to walk more than a couple of blocks without resting. A sudden and burning pain in his arm and chest led to an emergency surgical procedure, followed by three days in the intensive-care unit. He was a victim of coronary artery disease triggered by the stress of his family life.

TERRI PROBABLY FELT much more connected to Mayview than Meggan did to Western Psych, a reality that hit home quite jarringly early in 1992 when she learned that upon the occasion of her eighteenth birthday she would be transferred out of Mayview, perhaps forever, and into an adult facility—a prospect that terrified her. "I see the adults walking around here. It's so hard to believe that I could be like *them.*" She uttered the word with a queasy distaste.

I had initially scheduled a visit with Terri to say good-bye for a different and very exciting reason. Terri, I had been informed, was finally leaving Mayview for a wonderful new foster family—the same family who had taken in her older sister years ago, helped her through school, and eventually adopted her. This was Terri's surviving sister who was still in the Navy, stationed in California. The foster family had grown fond of Terri, wanted her to live with them and attend college in the fall at their expense. To Terri, this was her dream come true. A family. College. A chance to straighten out her life. By the time I visited Terri a month later, however, although she was leaving Mayview, the fleeting optimism for the future had faded into the dust of discarded dreams.

The family had come to visit Terri frequently and then had invited her home for weekends so they could get to know her better. The most important visit took place Christmas week, corresponding to a visit from her sister on furlough. Their reunion was exciting, but almost immediately a sibling rivalry emerged for the attentions of their foster family. "We fought all the time," Terri said. "Stupid stuff. If I chewed with my mouth open, she yelled at me. One time I took my medicine which makes me drowsy, and I fell asleep. Next thing I knew, she was screaming and yelling because I hadn't done some chore I had been asked to do. It got to be terrible."

Terri compounded the discomfort by announcing that she had decided not to go to college, at least right away, but to earn her GED and try to make some sense of her life. The family "didn't think that I would get anywhere in the future with just a GED. They said that if I decided not to go to college, then I couldn't live with them.

"Everything had been going so good," she told me, as we sat in a borrowed office, sipping Coke from cans. I had been made responsible for guarding the cans, making certain that Terri did not detach one of the tabs, which she could use to hurt herself. At this moment, Terri was on CVO (constant visual observation), which meant that she was never left alone. When she was in her room, an aide sat by her door, always watching. "Lately I have been seeing this guy standing in the corner. He just stands there, holding a knife. But when someone is sitting and watching me, he goes away." The man had tormented her in her dreams before, but not recently. He had returned to haunt her after the Christmas incident with her foster family.

After having fought with her sister for the entire week, Terri's nerves were so shattered by Christmas Eve that she reverted to her self-mutilating behaviors—and cut her wrist. Panicked, her foster family returned her to Mayview immediately. Later, when Terri tried to telephone, to apologize and explain, they refused to take her call.

She told her story haltingly, prompted by my questions. She was always open and relaxed with me and, oddly enough, amused by her bizarre and destructive behaviors, which she would often laugh about as she described them. Sometimes I couldn't help laughing with her. A smile appeared on her face when I asked her what she did in response to her foster family's rejection of her on the telephone. She blushed and giggled.

"I went out for a walk when it was snowing, and the maintenance people had put this rock salt down on the ground to melt the snow. I just picked up handfuls of the stuff and ate as much as I could before someone stopped me. Back in the dorm, I drank a bottle of fingernail polish remover which made me turn blue. And then I started to scratch myself." I reached over and lifted back the cuff of her sleeve to examine a large purple bruise. "Oh yeah, I burned myself on a heater," she added.

"Oh, my God," I said spontaneously, raising my brows and rolling my eyes. We both burst out laughing.

There was silence for a while, as we stared down at the desk and shook our heads, contemplating her plight. "None of this makes any sense," I told her. "It's . . ." I couldn't find a better word, so I used the one that had most easily come to me. ". . . crazy."

"I know," Terri agreed. "Everybody has been telling me that I am punishing myself for something other people have done to me. I don't feel like I am punishing myself, but maybe it's true. I guess I am an innocent bystander."

21

MY CONVERSATIONS WITH John VanDenBerg, Robert Friedman, John Burchard, and Jane Knitzer helped me to understand the vise of disorganization and overrestriction that renders the child mental health care system so ineffective and absurd. For four years, I have watched Daniel bounce from group homes to mental hospitals and back to the family from which he had been wrenched, from school to school, from one disturbing incident to another, including charges of theft, arson, and his own possibly self-created molestation. Based upon figures supplied by the state mental health office, and my own calculations, perhaps $2 million has been spent upon his care, treatment, and education. And yet, he can hardly read or write, add or subtract, remember the months in a year, or take care of himself any better than he could when I first met him. After all the resources expended upon psychotherapy and behavior modification, he was permitted to roam the streets endlessly, without purpose and direction. No psychiatrist regularly monitored his medications.

If anything, Terri's situation is worse than Daniel's—and gaining momentum in a rapid downhill slide. It's terrible enough living in an adolescent ward of a psychiatric hospital or in a group home, but kids will always look forward to a better future, even if it is unlikely or impractical. Once one is committed to an adult facility, it becomes much more difficult to fool yourself into believing that a more positive, happier life is possible.

And then there are the Scanlons. Other than George Orwell, Rod Serling, Charles Dickens, or of course, Kurt Vonnegut, who would have ever conceived of the notion that Americans in the 1990s, with the most advanced and expensive health-care system in the world, would have to relinquish custody of their own children with mental health problems in order to ensure their treatment? (And then discover that the treatment for which they have battled so desperately is inappropriate and ill-conceived?) A final blackhearted irony is to see your daughter virtually become a next-door neighbor living with a very well-to-do foster family, which is actually receiving the financial subsidies that were denied the biological family without relinquishing custody. A similarly ludicrous situation for, say, pediatric heart transplants or juvenile diabetes would precipitate mass protests. But because the issue is mental illness, a myste-rious and frightening malady we do not have the courage and compassion to confront, we turn the other way. Since we cannot see the demons of Daniel's and Terri's disorders, we pretend they are not there.

My scientist/clinician friends at Western Psych point out that very little traditional scientific research (with control groups) has been conducted to demonstrate the viability of the family preservation and individualized care models, although there do exist many positive and impressive anecdotal studies, such as the Burchards' AYI report. But there are similarly no scientific controlled studies that demonstrate that institutionalization is particularly effective. I agree that more studies should be launched in order to assess the overall effectiveness of all alternative child mental health care solutions, but we cannot afford to wait five years for the information to be gathered, the results tabulated and evaluated, before we act.

The time has come to take a daring chance by plunging headfirst into a new order in child mental health care. Seeing Daniel, Terri, and the Scanlons suffer so needlessly demonstrates the critical importance of initiating decisive and revolutionary action to save as many of these "damaged" kids as possible, before it is too late. It is true that solutions for universal societal ills stemming from burgeoning poverty (as in the case of much mental illness) must be confronted at the highest levels of government, as reports from the National Commission on Children and other prestigious groups have strenuously urged, but at the very least we can provide relief for many young people with mental health problems—today—simply by changing our approach and altering a failed philosophy.

As I write these words, I can't stop thinking about what might have happened if somehow, by some incredible miracle, John VanDenBerg had brought his individualized care approach to Pittsburgh. (In fact, John Burchard and Karl Dennis, an originator of the WrapAround concept, are currently implementing a nationwide effort to develop and evaluate WrapAround services.) Or what might have occurred if the Homebuilders family preservation model had been available to the Scanlon family.

How much suffering and misery might have been avoided if the Scanlons had received the respite care for which they were so desperate—just a way to get out of the house a couple of times a week for a quiet dinner without worrying about "World War III" at home? How would their lives have been altered if a caseworker had been available to help Meggan focus upon her studies after school, to help her go to sleep at a reasonable hour without disturbing her parents' privacy, and even to awaken her in the morning and help her prepare for school? It is quite possible that after a few months of such intense intervention, at a cost of $5,000 to $6,000, Meggan and her parents could have learned to handle their problems on their own. With such stability and support, perhaps the medications that Meggan had been taking, combined with Kenneth Stanko's considerable efforts in family therapy, would have been more fruitful. Western Psych and Ridgeview might have been inevitable destinations, but surely one needn't attempt the most drastic, last-resort problem-solving approach first.

Terri is probably more severely disabled than Meggan, but one can imagine the great potential of an individualized care plan to support and strengthen her life. When she was transferred from Western Psych to Ridgeview after her ECT trials, both Dr. Boris and Debbie Rubin lamented the inflexibility of the system. Terri needed to be slowly weaned from Western Psych and carefully, gradually, and intelligently introduced to the new world waiting in a more loosely structured facility like Ridgeview. Not only was Terri overly attached to Western Psych and

Dr. Boris, her history clearly indicated that she would do anything possible to sabotage herself.

But even by bending the rules, Dr. Boris could manage only to arrange a couple of preplacement weekends at Ridgeview before the drastic transfer. If Terri had been allowed to make the transition into Ridgeview at her own gradual pace and if a therapist had been assigned the pivotal and singular role of nursing and facilitating that transition, isn't it possible that Terri's placement would have been successful and on her eighteenth birthday, instead of being doomed indefinitely to an adult psychiatric facility, she might with therapeutic help have been able to transfer to an independent living situation? Maybe she would be going off to college—instead of an adult institution.

Similarly, what about Terri's difficulty with her sister and her foster family? There is nothing unusual about sibling rivalry—or in parents or guardians fighting with their children about their vocational and educational future. With individualized care and the crisis-counseling aspect of family therapy, isn't it conceivable that Terri's problems with her sister and her foster parents could have been worked out? No one at Mayview or in the CYS district responsible for Terri attempted to intervene with the foster family on Terri's behalf.

Later, I presented Terri's case to John VanDenBerg, who designed a theoretical "WrapAround" plan that might have helped bridge the gap between Mayview and Terri's potential foster family. "Terri has important strengths—a sense of humor, siblings, good hopes for the future—even though she has no basis in experience for them. She seems to respond to medication, except when her environment gets too scary."

VanDenBerg visualized a treatment plan beginning with the renting of a transitional apartment for Terri midway between Mayview and her potential foster home. Terri would be allowed to select and purchase her own bedroom furniture for the apartment, which would remain in her possession during any subsequent transfer. A favorite nurse from Mayview would live in the apartment with Terri for the first few weeks until one of the foster parents, who would have received special training in dealing with Terri, gradually replaced her. Terri would visit the foster home with increasing frequency. Within a couple of months, Terri would move into her foster home, along with an extra staff member who would be gradually phased out.

Terri would be provided with medication monitoring and regular psychiatric counseling. Foster parents would receive respite support. Terri's plan would cost at least $80,000 for the first year, according to VanDenBerg. The cost would be dramatically reduced in subsequent years, probably to less than $30,000. "Terri will try again and again to fight this plan; she will do whatever she can to get back into Mayview." Expect twelve to fifteen crisis episodes, VanDenBerg advised, before significant progress can be made.

VanDenBerg's suggestions for the Scanlon family begin the day of Meggan's second discharge from Western Psych, in consort with Dr. Stanko's therapy. Elizabeth and Tom would immediately receive a week's vacation, with child care provided for both children. A rotating live-in staff member would be employed to implement a consistent behavior management policy. A nearby apartment could be temporarily rented to which Elizabeth and Tom could retreat during especially difficult confrontations.

As Meggan's behavior improves at home, it might begin to deteriorate at school. The treatment team manager (perhaps Dr. Stanko) would meet regularly (daily, if necessary) with a coordinating teacher who would monitor Meggan's difficulties and act as a liaison to administrators and Meggan's other teachers. The school's commitment to Meggan must be as unconditional as that of her treatment team at home. She must not be permitted to engineer a suspension. A job in a local business would be arranged for Meggan and friends would be recruited and encouraged to visit. A regular link would be established between a favorite nurse at Western Psych and Meggan. Meggan should be permitted to return to Western Psych in the event of an emergency, but as with Terri, her stays should be brief and nonreinforcing.

VanDenBerg designed a similar WrapAround program for Daniel with respite support for Linda and a series of reinforcing rewards to persuade her husband, John, to become an active treatment team partner. I was also included on the team, as was Daniel's biological older brother—another related but relevent challenge.

It is significant to note that nothing VanDenBerg suggests is particularly creative or surprising; it's mostly a combination of common sense and old-fashioned family support and togetherness. And his plan certainly had no guarantee of working. But what struck home was that it hadn't been tried before. The system had been stretched in dozens of artificial directions, but the most logical possibilities, such as providing Terri with a transition from Mayview to a new destination, had never been seriously investigated.

Soon, Terri will close her eyes at Mayview a child, and awaken eight hours later an adult. She will pack her belongings, be put into a car, and be transported two and a half hours away, where she will be admitted into a long-term adult psychiatric facility. No one can deny the potential permanent devastation of such an experience. Terri, a kid who has never been able to make her own decisions and who has caved in at every sign of stress, will be expected to endure the most difficult transition of her life alone. It doesn't take John VanDenBerg to make us aware of Terri's needs. Sending her into such a tumultuous atmosphere without a well-formulated program to help her is not only ludicrous but immoral.

THE SAME WEEKEND I visited Terri at Mayview, Daniel's world crashed down upon him—one more time. It began when Daniel or someone resembling Daniel was seen stealing a car in his neighborhood. Daniel was questioned by the police and his mother. He denied having anything to do with the theft, but was enraged at his mother's suspicion. Tension had been increasing within the household over the months. Linda had been trying to exert control over Daniel, but he was flexing his muscles, exercising his own adolescent prerogatives to come and go and do what he pleased. The car-theft incident was the last straw for both mother and son. "I couldn't stand the sight of that woman anymore," Daniel told me. "I didn't want anything to do with her and I was sorry I had ever come home in the first place. I left the house and I swore I would never go back."

Daniel did what any kid in his particular circumstances would do. He had no family, no friends, no support system in his life, no training or preparation to care for himself even under the best of circumstances. He had never been able to focus upon his problems and think logically. His only option—the only action he knew he could take—was to appeal to the people who had made him so vulnerable and dependent in the first place.

Thus, he marched into the emergency room of the hospital nearest his home and said exactly what he, Terri, and all the other lost and desperate kids knew that the doctors, nurses, and social workers needed and maybe wanted to hear. He said he was depressed, suicidal, and homicidal. He wanted to kill someone with his gun. He didn't have a gun, but invoking one added impact and immediacy, Daniel told me later. A nurse wrote out his statements on a voluntary commitment form, which he confirmed, although he probably was unable to read them.

It is not clear where Daniel had hoped to go and what he imagined he could accomplish by making such statements. It isn't even clear that he had been serious about his intentions, but it was all he could think to do or to say. As it turned out, the system let him down one more time. Supposedly, there were no adolescent beds available at that moment in the county, not at Western Psych or ANI or anywhere else. And so, for lack of any other option, he was transferred to an adult facility with people two, three, and even five times his age. There was only one other kid in the unit, Daniel told me on the telephone a few days later, a boy who had been shot in the leg in the process of robbing a convenience store, and who kept banging his fist against the wall in irrepressible spasms of rage.

Daniel was all alone—again. The consulting child psychiatrist in the facility, who had just met Daniel, discontinued the antidepressants Daniel had been taking for the past five years and prescribed mood enhancers along with Haldol, which made him dopey and unfocused. "I'm all screwed up and I can't think," he said in a silly lilt. "I gotta get out of here, although I don't know where I want to go. This was a big mistake." So was going home to his mother, he admitted. "My mother couldn't take care of me." And in the jargon that he had come to know so well, he added, "The placement was entirely inappropriate."

But this was only the beginning of the next round of wretched horror stories. Although the adult facility was completely inappropriate, Daniel remained there for approximately six weeks before being transferred to a temporary shelter where he was scheduled to stay until a permanent placement could be found. Less than two weeks later, after having a fight with a fellow inpatient who had been acting out, Daniel was transferred to an adolescent ward of a local psychiatric hospital. Over the next three months, each time I came to visit, carrying my Pizza

Hut pizza, Daniel complained of memory loss from overmedication. He was gradually gaining weight. His behavior was bizarre, especially concerning where he would next be transferred.

Daniel said that he didn't care where he went—as long as it wasn't Mayview. He swore that he would never return to Mayview under any circumstances. Mayview was the end of the line, or so he said. Back where he started in a place he never belonged. One evening when I visited, he was profoundly depressed. "They want me to go back to Mayview," he said. "This is the worst moment of my life. I'm desperate. I can't go back there—or I'll die."

"Did you tell your doctor that you didn't want to go?" I asked.

"He won't listen to me." Daniel handed me a copy of the commitment papers he signed when he entered this facility. I was astounded to see that the doctor had noted that Daniel had specifically requested that he be sent to Mayview.

"It says here you want to go to Mayview," I told him.

"That's a lie," said Daniel. "I never said anything like that."

On my way out, I asked for a conference with the charge nurse, to whom I explained Daniel's abhorrence of Mayview. "This doesn't make sense," the nurse told me. "From the moment he arrived here, that's where he has been begging us to send him. He calls himself the 'Mayview man.'"

Daniel *did* return to Mayview, where he was often in the mood for confessing what had happened to him during his brief hiatus home— that horrific placement that CYS proclaimed so successful. With his street-gang friend, he had experimented with and "pushed" LSD, cocaine, marijuana, China White (a "designer drug" which had killed a number of people), and anabolic steroids. Indeed, his arms and legs had bulked up significantly with weight lifting and there were a number of purple broken veins on the biceps of both arms where he had injected the drugs. It was hard not to notice how heavy he was getting. On his seventeenth birthday, at five-foot-five, he weighed 215 pounds, more than twice his weight on his thirteenth birthday. Because he was constantly on restriction, Daniel devoted the entire spring and summer of that year—nearly six months in total—to video and TV watching. School was not in session. During his idle hours, he was obsessed by the thought of running away. He wanted to hide in an abandoned house in his old neighborhood, establish a drug-selling empire, and make his fortune.

Eventually, he was transferred to an independent living situation in which he shared a house with a counselor and a retarded thirteen-year-old boy, who was incontinent and prone to tantrums. It was a quiet, relatively controlled, and highly structured atmosphere. But only a few weeks later, Daniel called me to say that he was once again being transferred, this time to a foster family. "But you just got there," I said.

"That's right."

I couldn't believe it was happening to him again. Another broken attachment. "But that's crazy," I said.

"Lee," he replied softly, "only you and me seem to realize that."

Two months later, Daniel remained in limbo in the independent living situation. "When are you moving in with your foster family?" I asked.

He shrugged and stared down at his feet. "They are playing with my mind."

It is difficult to know exactly how many mistakes were made in caring for Daniel over the course of his life—and by whom. One cannot overlook the abuse and neglect of his early childhood and the biological predisposition to mental illness with which he was born, or the lack of unity and commitment to his cause by John and Linda when he had returned home. Linda had tried as hard as she could, but as Dr. Forrester had indicated at the court hearing, Daniel needed much more than Linda was capable of giving. She had not understood the extent of Daniel's difficulties and how ill-equipped she was to deal with such a troubled son—until it was too late. She was so blinded by anger and resentment toward CYS and any other authority figures in a society and system that had been so hostile to her that she was unwilling to accept any help they or anybody else had offered. She and John had even stonewalled attempts to permit counseling for Daniel after he was allegedly raped near my house, although he had repeatedly and immediately requested a therapist.

In retrospect, I believe that the rape was the beginning of the end of Daniel's short-lived and tragic reunification with his mother and sisters. At that point, rape or crisis counseling would have been helpful and might have served as a catalyst for a stronger, ongoing family therapeutic experience. Once again, I can't help thinking about the introduction of the individualized care concept at any of a number of junctures in Daniel's life. Most recently, instead of forcing Daniel to attend school in an inappropriate classroom, an electrician or a carpenter might have been hired to teach Daniel his trade. A special reading instructor, focusing upon manuals, diagrams, and other documents essential in electricity and carpentry, could have been provided.

What about a counselor to work regularly and intensely with his family *before* he was permitted to go home? Just because her husband refused to participate doesn't mean that a counselor could not have strengthened the bond between Daniel and his mom and eventually established the trusting foundation required to persuade other family members to join in. Was it fair to Daniel that he be denied the best schooling available in light of his behavioral problems and his learning disabilities because his mother's husband, a person of no relation, refused to be a part of the ancillary experience? Shouldn't the system have been flexible enough to accommodate the helpless victim?

As I look back on my life with Daniel, Terri, and Meggan, I clearly recognize that that is the key question. Why are children with mental health problems and those at risk forced to repeatedly suffer because of the incompetence and shortsightedness of the adults responsible for protecting them? Why can't we change the way we are doing things so that it becomes truly child- and family-centered? We need new and revolutionary leaders who will not be afraid to take chances, who are willing to confront and reject outmoded tradition. We must stop making the same old mistakes—and turn the mental health world upside down. Even if in the process we make new mistakes, we must use symbolic "shock therapy" to shatter the downward spiral of our damaged and defenseless children and provide a new and hopeful direction.

What happens in the next few years will determine the fate of not only 7.5 to 9.5 million mentally ill kids, but also their families and offspring—for untold generations. The Chilean poet Gabriela Mistral has written: "Many things we need can wait, the child cannot. Now is the time his bones are being formed, his blood is being made, his mind is being developed. To him we cannot say tomorrow, his name is today."

DANIEL

LATE THAT AUTUMN afternoon, I led two police officers back to the scene of the alleged molestation—the place to which Daniel had initially directed me. Daniel had told the police that the man had dragged him through the thick underbrush surrounding the abandoned building and molested him behind it. But the weeds and bushes revealed no sign of being trampled or disturbed, and later, the tests conducted by the hospital doctor were inconclusive. There were definite traces of semen on Daniel's shirt, but there was no evidence of penetration. Daniel could not explain to the doctor, the nurses, or the police investigators why he answered the telephone while walking toward the convenience store—or why he entered the man's car when he could have run in any direction, screaming for help.

During the following few weeks, the more people doubted and questioned the details and the logic of his experience, the more Daniel proclaimed its accuracy. "You may not believe me, and my mother may not believe me, and the police may not believe me," he told me, "but I know what happened. I don't care what anybody says. The man molested me. You don't know anything about it."

Daniel was right. I didn't know anything about it, and I guess the truth of the matter is that I really didn't want to. The situation was too

242

perplexing and too painful to dwell upon. Whether the rape had actually occurred or whether the entire incident was a creation of his own imagination, I have come to believe that it was a signal from Daniel—a cry for attention, help, and understanding to anyone who might listen. He felt himself slipping. Emotionally, he was circling the drain.

Rape constituted the loudest symbolic scream he could yell. And he had been partially successful. He had attracted the attention of the police, with whom he most desired contact, his mother, his big brother, his caseworker—all of the people in his life. We had all stopped dead in our tracks to look and to listen and to respond to Daniel, to be there for him during a brief time of need. But when the immediate crisis was over, the investigation completed and the new workweek started, everyone had returned to his or her own personal preoccupations. Daniel was still screaming for help, but we no longer had the time or the patience to listen. He was screaming into his future, which was as empty as his past.

Index

ADHD. *See* Attention deficit
  hyperactivity disorder
Admission decisions, 65–75, 77–79
  catchment areas and, 75
  health insurance and, 73, 74
  involuntary commitment and, 58,
    70–73, 77–78, 128
  search for suicide ideation in, 66–
    67, 70, 74–75, 78–79, 128
Adult psychiatric facilities
  children sent to, 238
  commitment to, 229, 233, 235,
    237
Aggression, 27
Alaskan Youth Initiative (AYI),
  205–10, 233, 234
Alcoholism, genetic link in, 27
Alexander the Great, 39
Allegheny Neuropsychiatric Institute
  (ANI), 128–29, 220, 233, 234
Alms, Lynn, 30, 153, 156, 157,
  158
American Journal of Psychiatry, 113

American Psychiatric Association
  (APA), 29, 55
Arbus, Diane, 39
Association for Children and Adults
  with Learning Disabilities, 83
Attention deficit hyperactivity
  disorder (ADHD), 27, 102,
    186, 187–94
  diet and, 187, 188–89
  Pelham's behavioral management
    program for, 190–94
  symptoms of, 101
Autism, 27, 30, 154–55
AYI (Alaskan Youth Initiative),
  205–10, 233, 234

Baughman, Annette, 68–73, 74,
  76, 77–81
Behavior modification, 14, 187
  in selection of psychiatric
    medications for children, 189,
    190–94